Healing Stories for Challenging Behaviour

Susan Perrow

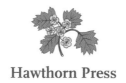

Hawthorn Press

Published by Hawthorn Press, Hawthorn House,
1 Lansdown Lane, Stroud, Gloucestershire, GL5 1BJ, UK
Tel: (01453) 757040 Email: info@hawthornpress.com
Website: **www.hawthornpress.com**

Cover illustration by Elizabeth Wang. Credit: God the Father loves us as His children with a tender and unfailing love, 2000 (oil on panel) by Wang, Elizabeth (Contemporary Artist). Private Collection/ © Radiant Light/ The Bridgeman Art Library. Nationality/copyright status: English /in copyright

Cover design and typesetting by Hawthorn Press, Stroud, Glos.
Reprinted 2021 by Henry Ling Ltd, The Dorset Press, Dorchester.
Printed on environmentally friendly chlorine-free paper manufactured from renewable forest stock.

The Fisherman, published with permission from the author, Elisabeth Aoko; *The Antelope, the Butterfly and the Chameleon,* published with permission from the author, Lucy Njuguna; *The Feather from the Lake,* published with permission from the author, Catherine Karu; *The Towel Poem* and *The Towel Story,* published with permission from the author, Emily Stubbs; *The Story of Silky Wriggly* and *A Story for Simon – Why the Sky is Blue,* published with permission from the author, Susan Haris; *A Ball of Wool,* published with permission from the author, Jane Dolahenty; *Child Star,* published with permission from the author, Alison Brooking; *Shimmer Wing* and *Never-Get-Enough,* published with permission from the author, Sandra Frain; *The Monkey Tree,* published with permission from the author, Jilly Norris. Please note that all stories that have been previously published by Immortal Books have had slight changes for this edition, and are included with the knowledge of Immortal Books.

British Library Cataloguing in Publication Data applied for
ISBN 978-1-903458-78-5
eISBN:978-1-907359-21-7

Dedication

For all children ... everywhere.

Acknowledgements

To my three boys, Kieren, Simon and Jamie, who have been intricately woven with my storytelling journey.

To my husband, John, whose support and love is more than I could ever have imagined.

To my grandchildren with whom I hope to share many stories.

To Nancy Mellon, Martin Large, Michael Moran and Matthew Barton who recognised the light of my storytelling and encouraged and helped me write this book.

To my long-time friend, colleague and mentor, Susan Haris, who taught me to 'never say no to a challenge'.

To all the children, parents and teachers in Australia and Africa who have inspired my writing, and sung and danced with me along the way.

Contents

Stories by Susan Perrow

Not published before:

'Cloud Boy'	The Beautiful Queen
Bored Baboon	Noisy Gnome Story
Whingeing Whale	Garden of Birds
The Secret of Easter	Jeremy and the Magic Sticks
Dishonest Dingo	Princess Light
Cherry Red	The Snail and the Pumpkin
Tembe's Boots	Anything New
The Little Girl Who Loved Flowers	Farmer 'Just Right'
Greedy Possum	Little Shell
The Frangipani Maiden	God's Garden
Pesky Pelican	Cranky Crab
Impatient Zebra	The Magic Stick
The Three Weaver Brothers	The Water Child
Mother Rabbit and the Bush Fire	Tidy Teddy

Published by 'Immortal Books'
in 'Gifts from the Sea' (1996, 2005):
A Little Boy went Sailing
The Grass Star Man

Published by 'Immortal Books' in 'Garden of Light' (2002):

Little Straw Broom	The Littlest Bubble
Restless Red Pony	Grandmother and the Donkey
Born to be King	Garden of Light
A Doll for Sylvia	The Pocket Knife and the Castle
Baby Bear Koala	Lindelwe's Song

Published by 'Immortal Books'
in 'The Knocking Door Tree Forest' Collection (2004):
Jaden and the Fairy Eggs
Strawberry Shy and Raspberry Wild
Pumpkin Munchkin

Stories transcribed/re-written by Susan Perrow

The Star Apple
The Old Woman and the Ants
The Magic Fish
The Invisible Hunter
The Story of Rhodopese
How Beetle Got Her Colours
The Three Billy Goats
The Enormous Nail
A Bag Of Nails
The Elves And The Shoemaker
Stream, Desert, Wind

The Doves and the Hyena
Benjie and the Turnip
Anansi and the Statue
Akimba and the Magic Cow
Anansi And His Shadow
Being Greedy Chokes Anansi
Anansi and the Birds
The Doves and the Hunter
The Squeaky Bed
The Little Clay Girl
The Frog and the Pail of Cream

Stories written by others

Ball of Wool Poem – Jane Dolahenty
The Towel Story – Emily Stubbs
The Fisherman – Elizabeth Aoko
The Feather from the Lake – Catherine Karu
The Antelope, The Butterfly & The Chameleon – Lucy Njuguna
The Sky's Blue Cloak – Susan Haris
The Story of Silky Wriggly – Susan Haris
Mother Moon – Alison Brooking
Never- Get- Enough - Sandra Frain, B.C.S, M.S.C
Shimmer Wing – Sandra Frain, B.C.S, M.S.C
The Monkey Tree – Jilly Norris

Stories written by others and summarised by Susan Perrow

The Brownies
Red Truck Story
Chameleon Story
Fly Eagle Fly

Foreword

Storytelling began its extraordinary revival throughout the world in direct response to wave after wave of electronic inventions. As our powers of listening and speaking have been spirited away into an array of mechanical devices, longing has awoken for more wholesome, direct communication. As if foreseeing cell phones, computers and text messages, storytellers began gathering to rediscover this neglected art. By the beginning of the 21st century, tens of thousands of people had heard the call: 'Be a storyteller; stand on your own two feet in the here and now; warm your heart and breath; hone your imagination; restore the speech that resounds throughout body and soul.'

Now, as televisions reign almost life-size in kitchens, living-rooms and waiting rooms, and printed materials heap up unread in every corner of the house, storytelling circles are meeting all over the world to experience a different kind of communication. An increasing number of parents, grandparents, teachers and community leaders are on a quest to reclaim their natural birthright as storytellers. As they rediscover and nourish whole sentences, plot lines and eloquent turns of phrase, much-needed warmth is flowing again heart-to-heart in homes, schools and every sort of meeting place.

As well as being an entertainer and an artist, the storyteller can offer healing. From time immemorial, the paths of storyteller and healer have intertwined. Even a one-minute, inspirational story can change both tellers and listeners for the better. A shamanistic impulse awakens as storytellers discover that imagination has infinite resources for picturing problems of every sort and bringing to light transformative wisdom that has been overlooked or suppressed.

As our new century began, a group of visionary social workers, educators and therapists decided to reach out to see who else was using storytelling as preventive medicine and to promote health. The response was resounding. Many people working with storytelling in all walks of life stepped forward. Ongoing conferences and alliances formed. Today a well-organised international Healing Story Alliance, based in the USA, is joined by storytelling alliances in the UK, Sweden, Australia and in many other countries around the world to support an oral tradition that restores joy and integrity to the spoken word.

As part of this growing movement, I was invited to Australia for the first time in 2006 to give a course exploring the effect of stories on body and soul. My journey unexpectedly took me to Byron Bay, where the author of this book invited me to stay with her. Modestly, Susan Perrow began to share with me her very extensive accomplishments as a storyteller and teacher. As her experiments and discoveries with storytelling gradually came to light from drawers and notebooks, I thrilled to discover how brilliantly she had been responding to the healing storyteller's call for many years. The book that you are about to read was born in the awareness that flashed between us then.

After many months of steady work, Susan Perrow's inspirational adventures with storytelling have grown into this inspiring book. I am confident that her wisdom, imagination and generosity will kindle the joy and healing power of storytelling within you. May these pages encourage you to speak healing words that help both children and adults to flourish.

Nancy Mellon, author of *Storytelling with Children*

Introduction

The Healing Light of Stories

When I first experienced the power of story as 'healing' for challenging behaviour – both in my own and other people's children – it felt as though a light had illumined the dark. As time went by, my parenting and teaching turned increasingly to such 'story lights' as I started interweaving wisdom tales from other cultures with my own story-making.

Many years later, while working as a teacher trainer in East Africa, I discovered a beautiful Kiswahili word that captured this illumined experience: 'ANGAZA' – 'to light up' …. Hadithi kwa kuangaza usiku – *Stories to light up the night.*

The aim of this book is twofold: to share these 'story lights' with you, and to help you create your own healing stories. Working with both modern and traditional tales, and many personal stories, the following chapters offer imaginative possibilities for transforming problematic behaviour and situations with children. They also provide teachers, parents, childcare workers and child therapists with a range of skills to create stories that address challenging behaviour.

Included in the text are eighty stories divided into different behaviour categories for easy reference – to work with directly, adapt, or use as models for creating your own tales. Brief notes precede each story, with an age guide and suggestions for use. The categories cover many kinds of commonly identified challenging behaviour, from dishonesty through laziness to teasing and bullying; everyday situations like 'tidy-up time'; experiences such as 'moving house'; or problems and difficulties such as 'separation anxiety', 'fear and nightmares' and 'illness and grieving'.

The range of selected stories and ideas are suitable for ages three to eight. However, stories often elbow their way out of the boxes we make for them. Sometimes a story written for a child may have a transformative effect on a teenager or an adult. Examples of this are shared through the book.

> It is easy to forget how mysterious and mighty stories are. They do their work in silence, invisibly. They work with all the internal materials of the mind and self. They become part of you while changing you.
> Ben Okri[i]

If you feel inspired to write your own therapeutic tales, the text provides a story-making model – a threefold framework of 'Metaphor', 'Journey' and 'Resolution' – to guide you. Based on a dictionary definition of healing – 'Bring into balance, become sound or whole', therapeutic stories for challenging behaviour or challenging situations are presented here as stories that help restore equilibrium or wholeness where behaviour is in some way out of balance.

In this story-making model, metaphors help build the imaginative connection for the listener, embodying both the negative, unbalancing, and the positive, rebalanced states. The journey itself builds the 'tension' as the story evolves, leading the plot into and through the behaviour 'imbalance' and out again to a wholesome, positive (not guilt-inducing) resolution.

Besides this framework, the book has chapters on age-appropriate stories, multicultural perspectives, props and presentation aids, and guidelines for the telling of stories. It is my hope, with some help from these sections, that you will feel encouraged to write and tell your own stories, and so perpetuate and develop age-old story traditions.

In many traditional cultures throughout human history, wise 'elders' have drawn naturally on metaphors and stories in their role as mentors and guides for the children in their tribes and communities. Using 'wisdom tales' to guide and invoke behaviour, they have tapped into children's imaginative reality and reached children in positive, affirming ways. This book encourages a revival of such use of metaphor and story.

How to use this book

My advice to readers is to begin at the beginning and, without too much analysis and questioning, simply dive in and follow my 'story journey'. Many personal anecdotes have been included here, hopefully to whet your appetite. Then you may wish to move to the third and fourth sections and read a few stories from different behaviour categories. When you feel you want to engage with the construction of these stories, and explore how to make up your own, return to the second section for help with 'Writing Therapeutic Stories'. Finally, when you are ready to tell a story, refer to the last section for tips on 'The Art of Storytelling'.

I have made no attempt to divide the resources into 'parent', 'teacher' and 'therapist' sections, since I believe there is so much overlap. A parent could gain ideas for tidying in the home from a teacher's story addressing lack of cooperation at group tidy-up time; a teacher could get inspiration from a story written by a parent to address dishonesty in the family; a therapist could both contribute to and learn from new ideas and metaphors for home and school situations.

Please remember that stories are not magic pills with powers to fix or heal all difficulties and challenges. Neither can there be a list of stories to suit every situation. Behaviour is relational and contextual. It can rarely be addressed in isolation. Each child exists and develops within an intricate web of relationships and environments – family, school, community and global. It is you, the practising reader, who is in direct touch with the relationships, context and individual characteristics of the children whom you parent, counsel and teach; you are best placed, therefore, to create stories for individual needs.

If this book achieves its main objective and inspires you to create healing stories for children, don't get stuck on expecting perfection. Your stories may have cracks, but – to quote Leonard Cohen, 'that's how the light gets in'. What is important is that you give it a go! The light that gets in through the cracks may be your best teacher.

> Ring the bells that still can ring; forget your perfect offering.
> There is a crack, a crack in everything – that's how the light gets in.[ii]

Healing Stories is the culmination of many years of practice, many years of 'giving it a go'. Compiling these pages has been both a struggle and a pleasure. The theoretical framework has taken much effort. The stories themselves, spanning more than thirty years of parenting, teaching and counselling, have flowed more easily onto the pages.

From several decades of running storytelling workshops and seminars, my general experience is that our inner 'storyteller' is once again seeking ways to unfold and shine forth. This book is a contribution to the universal revival of story in family, school and community life. I hope you will find treasures within these pages to help bring the healing light of story to the children in your care.
Susan Perrow, September 2007

SECTION ONE

MY STORY JOURNEY

1

From Dried Prunes to Juicy Plums: Why Use Stories?

Imagination and storytelling

A mother once brought her nine-year-old, potential 'prodigy' son to Albert Einstein and asked how her boy could further improve on his mathematics. Einstein replied 'Try telling him some stories.' The mother persisted in asking him about the maths issue. Einstein said 'Tell him stories if you want him to be intelligent, and even more stories if you want him to become wise.'

I first read about Einstein's views on stories and the imagination when I was a student teacher in the 1970s. As my favourite subject was maths, I felt drawn to his writings and was intrigued to read why a mathematical genius like Einstein placed imaginative thinking on a more important level than 'knowledge'. He argued that knowledge is limited to all we know and understand in the present, while imagination can embrace all there ever will be to know and understand. According to Einstein, imagination stimulates progress. Great inventions, he said, require an imaginative mind.

This was a new concept for me, and created my first link between stories, imaginative thinking and education. After passing my teaching degree at twenty-four I entered the workforce. Within six months I had my first experience of the power of 'story' on children's imaginations.

I was working as an assistant in a kindergarten in Sydney, Australia. In the weeks leading up to Christmas, the teacher decided to use a story from the Nutcracker Suite with its Christmas theme. She planned a visit to the class by the 'Sugar Plum Fairy'. Needing someone to dress up as the fairy, the teacher convinced me to trust her decision and take on this role. I remember first laughing at this idea, thinking that the children would be sure to recognise me, and that this would spoil the magical mood.

On the day of the festival I disappeared from class during playtime, went into the storeroom and changed into 'fairy' costume. I wore my mother's white satin wedding slip, carried a gold star wand in one hand, and a basket full of 'sugar plums' (nuts and raisins wrapped in red cellophane) in the other.

Meanwhile the teacher had gathered the 25 children around her, and at the appointed moment I nervously danced into the middle of the circle. The children sat in awe! As the teacher played some music from the story, I gave out a 'sugar plum' to each child. While I was doing this, one of the older boys, who had just turned six, reached out and touched my dress, saying with wide-open eyes, 'I've never touched a real fairy before!'

After changing back into my normal clothes, I emerged into the garden where the children were playing. Some of them were still carefully holding their 'sugar plums', not wanting to open them until their parents arrived. Others were eating them slowly and joyfully. When the children saw me, they cried out, 'Susan, where have you been, you missed the Sugar Plum Fairy!'

This left me with many questions. As the years passed and I became a mother of young children myself, my observations of the effect of stories on children's imaginations led me to further research.

To understand the breadth and depth of a child's imagination, I looked first at the difference between child and adult consciousness. I had studied child development during my training, and I understood that a child is not just a miniature adult. From direct observations of my own three boys and the young children in my classes there was a world of difference between us. The physical, emotional, social and cognitive differences seemed logically explained through maturation and development.

But what about the imagination? Unlike most other human qualities this power started out as vast and wondrous, then gradually shrank! I remember in my early childhood that imagination could transport me into the clouds (sometimes they became horses, or dolphins, or dragons); or take me over the hills and beyond our town (I would imagine following the train tracks that passed by our house, and being carried out into the big wide world on all sorts of adventures). This power could even admit me to the quivering, pulsating life of plants, flowers and insects in my garden. Back then I remember feeling that anything was possible and attainable – I was the world and the world was me! Years of so-called 'growth and development' later, I ended up as a young adult with limited imagination, needing to work on recovering my imaginative thinking. Many of my adult friends have had similar experiences. How could this be explained?

My quest for an answer has taken many years. I did not find it in texts on educational psychology or child development, but in the imaginative works of poets. The first insights that struck a deep chord in me came from Wordsworth's 'Intimations of Immortality'. Here he beautifully captures the journey of a child from ethereal worlds of spirit into birth, then through childhood, adolescence and on into adulthood.

From 'Intimations of Immortality' by William Wordsworth:

> *Our birth is but a sleep and a forgetting –*
> *The soul that rises with us, our life's Star,*
> *Hath had elsewhere its setting*
> *And cometh from afar –*
> *Not in entire forgetfulness,*
> *And not in utter nakedness,*
> *But trailing clouds of glory do we come*
> *From God, who is our home –*
> *Heaven lies about us in our infancy!*
> *Shades of the prison-house begin to close*
> *Upon the growing boy,*
> *But he beholds the light, and whence it flows,*
> *He sees it in his joy.*
> *The Youth, who daily farther from the east*
> *Must travel, still is Nature's Priest,*
> *And by the vision splendid*
> *Is on his way attended.*
> *At length the Man perceives it die away,*
> *And fade into the light of common day.*

This poem helped me form a more holistic picture of child consciousness. Rather than just 'advancing' from childhood to adulthood, there is also a loss. I have often felt that 'heaven lies about us in our infancy' when looking at a sleeping child – an experience of angelic presence, a sense of the divine. But these 'clouds of glory' fade, and, as Wordsworth laments: 'Shades of the prison-house begin to close, upon the growing boy' – until finally the 'vision splendid…fades into the light of common day'.

Could there, I wondered, be a way to keep this openness or vibrant connection from fading or shrinking?

I puzzled over this a long time. Then, just recently, I had a joyous discovery that gave me much encouragement as a storyteller. In his book *Matter, Imagination and Spirit,*[i] Owen Barfield, like Wordsworth, depicts two realities – the spiritual and the physical, the 'hidden' and the 'everyday'. But rather than abandoning us adults to this bare dichotomy he suggests a bridge between the two, a way of travelling from one to the other. This bridge or connection between matter and the spirit is the 'imagination' – beautifully depicted by Barfield as a rainbow bridge of imaginative activity. No doubt there are other ways to build this bridge – with prayer, meditation, music – but the idea of the 'imaginative' bridge rang wonderful bells for me.

These poetic illuminations helped me to understand why stories and fairytales speak so clearly to children, who are still in a much more dream-like stage, open to both physical and subtler, spiritual realities. Could truths contained in the rich realm of story reach children more directly, and in a way more in tune with their innate imaginative capacities? As adults, unless we have had an imaginative, story-rich education or have natural imaginative or creative gifts, it seems we have to work very hard to re-build our imaginative faculties.

When someone asked one of my sons at the age of six why he liked fairytales, he replied: 'Because they think about what I think about'. This childlike wisdom helped build another link in my chain of understanding – for a child the imaginative and spirit world could be as real as the physical, everyday world. Children seem to have the ability to cross back and forth on this bridge like butterflies. Most adults, on the other hand, struggle to take the smallest steps, like cumbersome many-legged caterpillars, from one realm to the other.

An elderly mentor once told me that the journey of a storyteller is a 'spiritual quest'. When I first heard this I wondered what the connection was between storytelling and spirituality. Now I understand why she believes this. Nourishing the imagination, stories can help us as adults to shed our caterpillar skins, metamorphose into butterflies and explore the gardens of 'hidden' reality.

Food for imaginative thought

A young doctor once attended a storytelling course I was running. In the introductory session, when it was his turn to say why he had enrolled, he told the group that he had been studying medicine at university for six years. As a result his mind, in his own words, felt like a 'dried-up prune'. He was hoping that storytelling would help make it a 'juicy plum' again, as he remembered it had been in childhood. Over the next few weeks, starting with a simple story of the life of a carrot (with carrot seeds and a real carrot as story props) he progressed to telling and writing imaginative tales. This same doctor now has a reputation for being wonderful with children. He keeps a story-bag in his surgery and to help relax his little patients he pulls out a story prop (a paper frog, a little doll, a shiny pebble…) and tells a story about it, gently easing the child into their check-up or injection.

In our busy adult lives it is easy for our imagination to 'dry up'. Like a muscle, it can atrophy from lack of use and may need exercises to build it up again. My secondary education focused on the sciences and rational thinking, and my shrinking imagination was rarely sparked by my teachers. As an adult I now feed my imagination through reading and writing poetry and stories. The students who enrol in my Storytelling unit at Southern Cross University, Australia, are advised to read a children's story every day of the term. If your imagination also feels like a 'dried-up prune', I suggest you start by choosing ten stories in this book and reading one each day. Although they are written primarily for children, you may find the metaphors and imaginative journeys feed your adult soul. If this is of benefit, I suggest you continue reading more stories, whether for children or adults. Fantasy novels like the 'Lord of the Rings' are another rich source of food for the imagination. It may also help to participate in a storytelling or writing course, and attend storytelling sessions.

The natural world can also be a wonderful source of inspiration. When I am pondering ideas for a story, I find that some of my best ideas come from nature. Walking through the bush or along the beach, sitting in the park or in the garden: these experiences have fed my imagination whenever I have 'writer's block'. Even housebound, I found that looking out through my window at the branch of a tree, with its patterned bark, budding leaves and silver raindrops, helped inspire a story idea.

Nature has the potential to relax and cleanse us, to strengthen and nurture us – in fact to reconnect us with ourselves. Especially when writing stories for young children, I find I need to bathe in nature's wonder and beauty on a regular basis to keep myself open to the wonder and beauty of life.

Scepticism and self-doubt

A common barrier to imaginative thinking in adults can be scepticism about the importance and relevance of stories to modern life. When I approached the Dean of Research at the local university about a scholarship for a research project on storytelling, his first response was to laugh at me; but then he challenged me to prove this was a real subject for research. It was a satisfying moment several years later to have him shake my hand at my Masters Graduation! His scepticism had slowly changed to genuine interest and the university soon added Storytelling to their list of subjects.

In my courses I meet scepticism on a regular basis. Once a psychologist/parent, who was attending the course asked to share an experience with the group. She told us how ridiculous she had thought all this 'story and imaginative stuff' was, and being a science student she had decided to put it to 'empirical' test. The previous week she had been in the park with her children. Near the swings she had overheard a grandmother having a fierce debate with her young granddaughter. The grandmother wanted the child to put the safety belt across the swing and the child kept refusing. So grandma wouldn't push the child and the child sat on the swing crying. Grandma was telling her that if she didn't put the belt on she might fall out, break an arm and end up in hospital, and her mother would be very cross.

The sceptical mother recalled an unusual creative flash while searching her mind for an imaginative rather than head-on approach. She asked the grandmother if she could help. Receiving permission, she looked at the little girl and said, 'Did you know that this swing has a magic sash, and if you tie it up it turns you into a princess and takes you swinging up high. Shall I tie it up for you'. The little girl stopped crying, looked up at her wide-eyed and nodded YES. So the surprised and no longer sceptical mother tied up the safety belt, grandmother started to push the child on the swing and the confrontation melted away.

Often people's scepticism is coupled with self-doubt about their own creative abilities. A father had been struggling to teach his four-year-old son to pee straight into the toilet and not all over the top and sides. After a session on the creative power of metaphor, he tried working with the simple visual word 'waterfall' (instead of the abstract word 'straight'). The father reported that the boy immediately took up the challenge to make an uninterrupted waterfall into the loo – every time he needed to go! The father was amazed at the result of a one-word change, and very chuffed at what he called his 'first creative achievement'. From this simple playing with metaphor, the father went on to make up stories at bedtime for both his son and daughter. He later commented on the positive bonding that resulted from this, coupled with his enhanced creativity.

Most teachers and therapists who attend my story-making work-shops respond with a resounding NO when asked if they think they could write a story before the day is over. Three to four hours later, their imaginations 'juiced' with many story examples, and with a framework to guide their ideas, they are usually surprised by the positive results.

Even African teachers, born and raised in a storytelling culture, frequently reveal this self-doubt. My focus for my Masters Research was informed by this – how could I, as a storyteller from a non-storytelling background, find ways to help African teachers 'wake-up' their cultural storytelling skills? One way was to encourage discussion and trigger memories through the power of story itself. In the training modules in Cape Town, after struggling to get a group discussion going, I decided to tell a simple story about a tree that was once tall and healthy with strong roots, and then through lack of care grew stunted and weak, and lost its leaves. These images helped the participants to recall childhood memories from their own 'story tree'. It encouraged an older woman to sit on the floor and demonstrate how her grandmother used to play the 'uhardi' at story time (a stringed musical instrument made from a dried gourd). From this beginning the memories and the stories really started to flow, and it was easy to build up a picture of the present 'story tree' and possibilities for its future. The story and the simple imagery of the tree inspired the women to talk. The session was much more fruitful than the previous one, when I had asked for memories of childhood and no one in the group wanted or was brave enough to speak. This discussion (which ended up filling two sessions) helped reconcile the group with the storytelling culture of their past; some storytelling skills, especially in the older women, were renewed; and a future enthusiasm for storytelling, both cultural and multi-cultural, was generated.

Another instance occurred when I asked a more experienced group in Cape Town to write and present a story of their own. Only three of the ten women came with their homework. The ones without stories walked in with heads down and very upset. 'It's too hard, Susan, we can't do it' they complained. I placed a chair at the front of the room, sat on it, and shared one of my own stories as a warm-up. Then the three women with homework shared their stories, with much prompting from me. By the time they had finished, the atmosphere in the room had completely changed. The three storytellers were feeling very proud of themselves. Then two more women jumped into the story chair and told stories that they made up on the spot. The women were convinced that the story chair had a special power, and together we adorned it with coloured ribbons. The following week the other five women arrived, insisted on sitting in the marked chair, and all proceeded to tell wonderful traditional stories.

'Born to be King'

A personal example of pushing through self-doubt is an experience that challenged my abilities as a therapeutic storywriter. On my first visit to East Africa I worked for an outreach teacher training centre. While running their storytelling module in Nairobi, I was asked by a young Kenyan mother for help with her son who had been sexually abused by his ayah (nanny) at the age of three. The boy had contracted a sexually transmitted disease as a result of this abuse. For several months, while the medication took time to work, it was extremely painful for him to pass urine. When I met the mother, the child was six years old, the disease was cured at a physical level, but at an emotional level the fear of the pain remained. He needed continual support to be able to go to the toilet – his mother needed to sit with him, sing to him and read to him until he could relax enough to let go…

Now that her son was ready to begin full-time schooling, the mother was desperate for something to help him overcome his fears. Could a story help, she wondered?

This question put me into humble shock, as I had been teaching about the 'healing' power of story and yet had never had to work with this kind of challenging situation. Of course, I wanted to help if I could, but I wondered if I had the skills and understanding for such a task. After all, I was not a trained psychologist. But I decided to give it a try. For the next few nights I didn't get much sleep – would-be storywriters be prepared for the midnight birthing of stories!

My first request was to meet the child. The mother arrived with a tall, proud and handsome brown-skinned boy by her side. When I saw him I thought that he looked like a young prince. Trusting my intuition, I said to the mother (out of the boy's hearing) that I felt the story should be about a prince who was 'Born to be King'. I was concerned, though, that kings and princes were not such a strong part of African culture. Her reply was that her son's favourite stories were about kings, queens and castles.

I now had my starting point. The next night I stayed up scribbling on a notepad in the dim light of many candles. Working with my framework of metaphor, journey and resolution I wrote

'Born to be King' (see page 230) and gave the mother a copy before boarding the plane back to Australia. The resolution was clear for me – the boy needed to find inner strength and confidence. Briefly, the journey would flow from the sunlight into the dark castle and back out into the sunlight. The obstacle and helping metaphors were many (see chapter on 'Writing Therapeutic Stories'). Two months later the mother's email to me confirmed the therapeutic success of this story. It was also wonderful encouragement for me to continue pursuing a path of therapeutic story work.

Listing reservations

At this early stage in the book, it is quite natural to expect you to have questions of your own about the value of stories and storytelling for children. Before reading any further it may help you to review the list below of five common reservations often expressed by workshop participants. Tick what applies to you, then add any more of your own.

☐ I am not a creative person

☐ I could never think up metaphors and imaginative ideas with children

☐ I could never write a story

☐ The challenging behaviours I am facing with my child/ children could never be addressed by an imaginative approach

☐ I am not convinced that stories have 'healing' potential

☐ ....

☐ ....

☐ ....

I suggest you check back with this list after finishing the book.

The next two chapters continue my personal story journey by documenting the effect of stories on my family and professional life. By including personal anecdotes and experiences I want to encourage you with examples of the tangible healing power of stories. Although I have divided these into stories for parenting situations, and those from the field of teaching and counselling, I encourage you to read both chapters, no matter what your occupation, as all areas of story experience with children can provide useful ideas.

[i] See reference section

2

Weaving Stories into the Family Fabric

The light of stories has woven many shining threads through the fabric of my family. In this chapter I share examples that have coloured and strengthened family life from the time when my three boys were very young through to their primary school years and beyond. To help with writing these experiences, I 'interviewed' my sons, Kieren, Simon and Jamie, at their respective adult ages of 29, 28 and 26. Their memories merged with mine, and are published with their permission. It is my hope that this sharing of experiences will help inspire you to interweave stories into your own family life.

Influenced by my storytelling experiences as a teacher (see next chapter), I entered parenting with a strong sense of the importance of stories for healthy child development. I continually gathered storybooks for my children from second hand bookshops, fairs and libraries. The collected stories expanded and grew as the boys developed – from nursery and nature tales, to folk and fairy tales from many cultures, myths and legends, and then, in their teens, biographical stories on explorers and adventurers (for more on story 'genres' see Chapter Six).

During the boys' younger years, our story bedtime ritual was one of my favourite parenting activities. Although most days I would find myself quite tired by the evening (especially during my single-parenting period), reading or telling stories was a soothing and re-energising experience. And if I was totally exhausted I could rely on some rhythmical and humorous ballads to bring me back to life…

The Owl and the Pussycat went to sea, in a beautiful pea-green boat …

Or

Christopher Robin had wheezles and sneezles …

This last poem in the AA Milne series[i] was a wonderful resource if any of the boys were unwell. I would sit on the end of their beds and read this aloud – the humour helped to lighten the situation a little. Another favourite from this series was 'The King's Breakfast' – a long story in rhyme about a king who wanted a 'little bit of butter' for his bread. It was an excellent one to recite as a way of changing the subject if the boys were arguing at the breakfast table!

Slowly the boys outgrew stories and poems read by me (and recited at the table) and moved on to devouring books by themselves. Reading books was a much more frequent activity in our home life than watching TV, and the positive effects of this was continually noted by their teachers. One of my boys won a competition once on the theme of 'Why Are Books Better Than TV'. Simon began his essay with 'I hardly have time to write this as the storybook I am reading is so exciting …' The prize was a book voucher of course.

The helping Brownie

When my oldest boy was seven, I received a remarkable and unexpected gift through the power of a story.

Simply entitled 'The Brownies', it was the next story to read to Kieren at bedtime. Taken from a collection of 'Golden Pathway' storybooks, the extra story was sometimes a treat for him once his two younger brothers had fallen asleep. 'The Brownies' injected a healing boost of energy and joy into my then difficult life as a mother of three young children.

The Brownies story was about two boys whose mother had died and whose father was struggling to raise them on his own. To do this he needed to work in his job during the day and do all the cooking and cleaning at night and early in the morning.

One day Grandma came for a visit and the oldest son asked her why his father was always so cross and unpleasant. Grandma replied that it was probably because the Brownies hadn't come to live in the house to help him do his work!

The boy wanted to know where he could find the Brownies to invite them back to the house to help do the work and make his father happy. Grandma replied that only the wise old owl in the forest knew where they lived. Then Grandma went home.

That night the boy had a restless sleep, and eventually decided in the dark hours of the early morning to go into the forest to find the wise old owl. He crept out of the house and along the forest path, and when he found the owl he told him his problem and asked where the Brownies lived.

The owl told him to follow the path back to the lake, stand on the edge of the water in the light of the moon, then say the following riddle to himself. He assured him that when he did this and solved the answer to the riddle, he would find out about the Brownies.

> *Twist me and turn me and show me the elf,*
> *I look in the water and I see …*

The boy did this and of course saw his reflection. Straight away he knew that he was the one who should be the Brownie doing the jobs. He crept back to the house and while it was still dark he set to work, cleaning the kitchen, preparing the fire and sweeping the floor. Just as it was getting light, he crept back to his room. He lay in his bed listening to the joyous cries of his father who had reached the kitchen and was so happy to find his work had been done – 'Oh happy day, the Brownies have come to stay!'

I only read the story to Kieren once. The next morning I woke in the dark to a scratching kind of sound coming from the bathroom.

My first thought was that I had left the window open and a possum had come in and fallen into the bathtub. I climbed out of bed and made my way up the hall. On turning the corner to go into the bathroom I felt utter amazement. There was my seven-year-old son, kneeling in the bath, with a tub of Ajax cleanser in one hand and a nail-brush in the other hand, scrubbing away, backwards and forwards …

I crept back to bed, feeling absolutely astounded and elated and yes, as in the story, very happy. I lay there for twenty minutes – Kieren was already showing signs of 'perfectionism' at his young age of seven, and was obviously eager to give the bath a really good clean. Finally I heard him creeping back to his room.

'I'll play out the story,' I thought, so I left my bed and reached the bathroom, announcing in quite a loud voice, 'Oh happy day, the Brownies have come to stay!' This was very easy to say as my bath was gleaming in the early morning light, and cleaning bathrooms was always last on my list of household tasks. I then went into the kitchen to start breakfast chores and when Kieren joined me a few minutes later he didn't say a word and neither did I. He just glowed with joy and so did I!

For the next two weeks Kieren woke in the dark and played out the Brownie story. Every morning he would attempt a new kind of task, but obviously was running out of ideas as after a while he just kept scrubbing the cupboard doors in the kitchen. As I was worried that the paint was going to get scrubbed off, I started to leave hints for new jobs … putting my shoes on the cupboard at night with the shoe brush and polish next to them … leaving some dishes in the sink to be washed in the morning …

We never spoke about this, and a few months later, after a particularly busy day, I slumped down in my chair and said, within earshot of Kieren, 'Oh how I wish the Brownies would come back to help again'. Well they did, but only for a few days, and then it was never mentioned again. I had to be very careful not to put too much pressure on this little worker.

To this day I will never know why or how this story had such a deep effect on Kieren. Was I perhaps the cross parent like the father in the story? Or did solving the riddle make a deep impact on this young boy? Certainly the story contained a remarkable journey for any listener. Instead of grandma or the wise owl telling the boy he needed to help his father, the boy had to discover this for himself. Many years on, when Kieren was in his late twenties, I pulled out the story and we chatted about his memories of these events. Interestingly enough, he only had vague memories of the story, but he certainly had strong recollections of doing the 'Brownie' jobs and his delight in keeping them secret.

Car tales and tangled knots

Children often have to be buckled into the back seat of a car for a long distance trip. Anyone who has lived in the vast continents of Australia and Africa will understand the amount of travelling hours that children have to sit still for.

As well as utilising various car games and car crafts that I had in my 'parent resource kit', driving for hours on end gave a chance for me to practise storytelling. I started with my favourite ones from childhood, for the practical reason that I would be able to remember most, if not all, of the story. I remember feeling quite nervous the first time I tried this, but clutching the steering wheel and staring straight ahead gave me some kind of confidence. The quietness in the back seat as the listening kicked in certainly encouraged me to continue.

On these long trips, the general healing power of storytelling influenced all of us. Three usually very active boys entered into active imagination and forgot, for the duration of the stories, to wriggle and tease and fight. And I would arrive at our destination less haggard and harried. When I shared this with an older friend she said, 'I know all about this. I learnt it from my grandmother. When I used to take my children mountain climbing I would 'story' them to the top and back down again'.

I have since read about this wisdom in the culture of the Bushman peoples of Southern Africa. They can wander the desert for many days, 'storying' their children along, telling tales about the hill in the distance, the rocks in the gully, the evening star rising over the sand dunes…

A similar sitting-still situation would arise when there were tangled knots to be brushed out of hair, or the constant 'nits and lice' check that came with living in the sub-tropics of Australia and in the humid climate of coastal Africa. I had learnt a strategy from watching African mothers spending hours braiding the hair of their young children. They kept them still by telling stories!

Quite often, the power of humour helped here. A niggle-naggle-knot-man was created to help these 'sitting' situations. He had various adventures that were sometimes made up by the child himself, or with ideas prompted by one of my poems:

First he's here, then he's there, but can you see him anywhere?
The wind blows him here, the wind blows him there,
The wind sometimes blows him into your hair,
The fishermen find he's been into their lines,
He's into the sewing threads all the time!
First he's here, then he's there, but can you see him anywhere?

With the nits and lice checks, it also helped to work through different versions of a 'naming' game that I remembered from my childhood. On the hill behind Tamworth, the country town that was my birthplace, I would sit in a large pepper tree with my friends and we would rename everything and everyone we could think of who lived in the town below:

RIVER bombiver stickeliver fifiver,
Fifiver stickeliver that's how you say RIVER!
JASON bombason stickelason fifason
Fifason stickelason that's how you say JASON
MRS SMITH bombith stickelith fifith
Fifith stickelith that's how you say MRS SMITH!

My boys loved using this as a chance to name all the other children in their class who also might have nits. When we ran out of children's names, we moved onto their teachers' names (they delighted in this!). Then, if more time was needed, we moved onto the objects in the room and outside the window. This would allow for plenty of hair-checking time.

Travelling through the wardrobe

Reflecting on the joys and trials involved in raising three sons, I am struck by the 'balancing' effect of their rich diet of nature and folk tales on their choices of play and recreational activities. Alongside the typical 'boy' weapon play with bows, arrows, guns and spears, and their sporting interests in skateboarding, cricket, football and surfing, there was always plenty of time spent on travelling 'through the wardrobe' into vast realms of imaginative play.

Recent discussions with all three have shown that these times formed some of their happiest memories. The local creeks were explored and re-explored for magic crystals, pirate hideouts were constructed in rock caves on the beach front, and miniature houses with intricate rooms and pathways were built in back corners of our garden for the 'little folk' to live in.

A strong memory of my middle son, Simon, concerns these little houses. When he was eight years old, we moved from our rented home to our 'bought' home. The first thing he did when we arrived with the furniture, was to lead his brothers out into the backyard and quickly build a new house for the fairies to move into – they were convinced that the fairies had followed the furniture truck!

The three boys also have special memories of the 'knocking-door tree' forest near my kindergarten (see next chapter), with the magic doors in the trees. Many years later, my youngest son and his friends spent an evening revisiting this forest to celebrate a twenty-first birthday.

Imaginative play and the 'little folk'

Throughout the boys' childhood I encouraged their imaginative play by providing simple resources. I saved large cardboard boxes and timber off-cuts for den building, and old clothes for dressing up. At garage sales I found hammers and digging picks for crystal hunting, and always tried to leave a good part of the garden 'untamed' for hiding places, tree houses and magic buildings for the 'little folk'.

For fear of it becoming sentimental, I was careful never to prompt any talk about 'fairies' or 'nature spirits'. But nor was it in the least discouraged. In fact I found myself listening to the boys' comments with intense curiosity. At a young age, my son Simon used to describe in limited, three-year-old detail the fairies that lived, alongside the monkeys, in our garden in South Africa. He would come and sit next to me on the grass that sloped down to the forest and chat away about what he could see. I was in awe at what I was hearing, and was very careful never to judge or label what he was sharing with me. These moments are still sacred memories – when a child's imaginative perception enriched my own.

As a child I am convinced that I could see 'dancing spirits' in the garden. I don't remember them looking like the typical fairies found in children's picture books, but more like dancing balls of light with vague faces and limbs. Because of these memories, combined with further reading on nature spirits and elemental beings,[ii] I have never questioned the existence of the 'little folk' immortalised in myth, legend, and children's stories. I am sure that as a young child I was seeing some of these 'beings'.

I could also see 'things' in the dark. My memory of this is quite clear. My older brother and I used to lie in bed and discuss what we could see, and more often than not we saw similar things. One night I saw an extremely scary shape in the doorway and cried out for my parents. The response was very disappointing – my father scolded me for talking nonsense, and told me to go to sleep. I never mentioned my 'sightings' to any one again, and yet the memory of these things stayed with me.[iii]

It may be hard for adults to engage with this realm of childhood perception, but it is nevertheless often a reality for children, and something of course which comes alive in many folk and fairytales. Rather than insisting that children see the world as we do, we can learn from them something we often forget – that nature is alive and ensouled, full of dynamic energies and vital, often unperceived realities.

Imaginative family traditions

When my eldest lost his first tooth, the current tradition as practised by families in our neighbourhood was to replace the tooth with a $1 or $2 coin. I thought about this and the materialistic basis of such a tradition, and decided to try something simpler and more imaginative. Instead of a dollar coin, the tooth fairies left a tiny shell instead. The comment made by my excited six-year-old boy in the early hours of the morning still rings in my ears – 'I knew the *real* tooth fairies wouldn't leave money!'

This seal of approval from an innocent child started a simple family tradition – for each tooth lost a natural treasure was left in its place (a shell, crystal, feather, etc). As an end to this was needed eventually, a special treasure box was left out with the seventh tooth, with a note suggesting its use as a home for the accumulated treasures. Decades later these little boxes, with their simple contents, are still kept as treasured memories.

An imaginative approach was also used to solve the question for my youngest – 'Is Santa really true?' This is a common question for families with younger children who hear comments from their older siblings who have outgrown such beliefs. One Christmas I sensed this was starting to happen in our household. Jamie was still at the tender age of five. I told a bedtime story to his older brothers to try to help the situation. This story was about Santa being a 'giving spirit' that enters children when they are old enough to be able to make their own gifts. They were so inspired by this that they set to work writing a list of every relative and distant family friend they could think of. Then a multitude of presents were made, wrapped and put under the Christmas tree – packets of hand-made cards, pots of jam, candles, bookmarks, etc. Needless to say, Jamie stopped hearing anything negative about Santa! Two years later he was also ready to hear about the 'giving spirit'.

I recently heard from a friend of mine, who grew up in a German/Serbian family of ten children, that her mother used a tradition of bringing home a special cake with each new baby. The cake was a light sponge with jam and cream, unlike any other kind of cake the children were used to eating. The children waiting at home were told that it was 'cake brought by the new baby from heaven'. They all looked forward to this, and greatly treasured the eating process (my friend said she would take several days to eat her piece!). In this way, each new child was received by the rest of the family in awe and wonder. My friend has no memory of ever being jealous or resentful of each new baby joining the family.

It is interesting to research and reflect upon the wisdom of family traditions and practices. Parents may gain imaginative insights from discussions with their own grandparents and great grandparents. My own grandmother, of strong Yorkshire stock, thought that if a child fell and hurt her knee,[iv] or was upset about something, then the best thing to do was to carry on working while singing a song with many verses. If, at the end of the song, the child was still upset, then it might be significant enough to attend to. My grandmother felt this approach was so effective because the imaginative content of the song usually captured the child's interest and helped her forget about why she was upset.

Poetry and creativity

As well as encouraging imaginative play and traditions, a rich diet of stories and poems has given the three boys a significant sensitivity to language. Since their early teens, they have enjoyed writing poetry, especially for special events. Over many years, a poem from one or more of my boys has been the main gift for my birthday. I keep a small treasure chest at home full of these loveliest memories.

My youngest son has recently decorated the walls of his flat with his travel photos and snippets of poetic writing, and his spirited approach to life is imbued with creativity. My middle son has a sensitive talent for writing and presentation. At a recent community event, he had the audience almost in tears as he described his life story viewed through his love of shell collecting.

My eldest, now touring the world as a professional surfer, often brings poetic metaphor into his articles submitted to surfing magazines. This pro-surfer proposed to his wife in a most creative way. He took her to the beach at sunrise and drew a heart in the sand for her to stand inside. Then he dived into the ocean and surfaced in front of his beloved lady with a sparkling ring in his hand … an engagement inspired by fairytales!

Bottles and bubbles

My first experience as a parent story-maker arose from an unusual stimulus. Up to this time I had always read or told other people's stories to my children.

Jamie, at three years old, hated having his hair washed, and I mean 'hated' with a capital H! Because it was such a traumatic experience for both of us, hair washing day, that had been a matter of course for his two older brothers, was put off as long as possible for Jamie. Finally my pride as a parent would take over, and I would try to sneak the hair washing into general bath time, but inevitably tense periods of loud screaming would ensue.

It was during one of these screaming sessions that I had a brilliant idea, although the credit for the brilliance should really go to the manufacturer of the baby shampoo. Instead of the usual bottle-shape, this particular manufacturer had chosen to package the product in a bottle shaped like a bear.

As I picked up the shampoo bottle, a crazy story started to race around my head, and eventually found its way out of my mouth and into Jamie's ears. If you are thinking I must have screamed the story, you are right! But only for the first few sentences, for as Jamie's ears opened the screaming stopped.

And so the simple story of Shampoo-the-Bear was born. Shampoo-the-Bear had countless adventures as he travelled through the forest, along the river, and into many towns. Everyone he met on his way would greet him with a friendly hello... but every time Shampoo-the-Bear opened his mouth to say hello back, bubbles would come out instead of words.

Shampoo-the-Bear totally transformed hair-washing time. In fact Jamie wanted to hear more and more stories about this remarkable character, and, for a while, hair washing was happening almost every other day. Of course the stories could only happen at hair washing time – I needed to open the bottle first before a story would come out – 'parent wisdom' practised here! For the times between, the bottle was kept on a very high shelf.

'Cloud Boy' wins a healing victory

One of my most difficult times as a parent was when my two older boys were at school and my youngest still had a year to wait. This could have been wonderful for quality time together, but because Jamie was born wanting to be number one in the family, he often could not accept being the youngest – especially in this last year before he went to school. Every morning when Jamie's brothers left to catch the bus, I had to draw on all my creative talents to distract him from getting upset and angry. And I must confess that my patience and creativity were wearing thin.

To add to this difficulty, Jamie's fifth birthday was coming up, and he desperately wanted a 'Masters of the Universe' warrior doll for his special day. This doll was sold to advertise the television show of the same name. It was made from grey rubber and had scars on its face and weapons at its belt. Jamie always prefaced his request by saying, 'All my friends have one!' Yet as a reasonably protective mother I wanted my son to have a less aggressive doll to play with and sleep with.

One week before his birthday I found a soft cuddly doll in a craft shop that reminded me of Jamie – it had a lovely petite face, white-blond hair and a little blue suit – Jamie's favourite colour. Jamie will love this, I thought, and I promptly purchased it and wrapped it for his special day. But on the morning of his birthday, when Jamie unwrapped a doll that was not the expected 'Masters of the Universe' version, he was so angry he threw his present on the floor and stormed out of the room.

Without giving too much detail, the next few weeks could be numbered amongst the most unbearable in my parenting life. Jamie was so angry with me! Yet I was determined not to give in to the commercial pressure that tries to invade our homes and private lives in so many insidious ways. A stalemate had developed, and just when there seemed no solution, I decided to try to heal the rift with a story – one inspired by the little doll that now lived in my bedroom cupboard.

For three nights, as Jamie was falling asleep, I stood by his top bunk and in a very nonchalant way, started to talk to him about a little child called Cloud Boy. I had to do this in quite a casual manner. Jamie had been very reluctant to join in any of our family rituals, including bedtime story, since his traumatic birthday.

Cloud Boy was a child who lived in the clouds in his cloud home, slept on a soft cloud bed, and ate cloud pancakes for dinner. Cloud Boy had hair the colour of white clouds, and wore a suit the blue of the sky. For a long time, Cloud Boy was very happy living up in the sky all by himself.

But one day his cloud home floated close to the earth and he could see lit-tle children, just about his size, playing in the fields and the gardens in the world below. Cloud Boy then decided that he wanted to come down to the world and have a friend to live with and play with. Every day he would travel across the sky in his cloud home, over the tops of the forests, along the rivers and over the mountains ... all around the world. He was looking for a friend who would play with him and look after him ...but where could such a friend be found?

By the third night, Jamie had forgotten his reluctance to engage in the bedtime ritual, and was showing great interest in this simple story. On this night the story had ended with the open question, 'Where could such a friend be found?'

Once Jamie was asleep, I crept into his room and stretched a long piece of white muslin to hang under his top bunk. I then carefully placed the little doll into the 'cloud' within full view of the ladder that Jamie would be climbing down the next morning. Later that evening I crawled into bed, not knowing if my story was going to help or make a change, but at least knowing that it had engaged Jamie's interest at bedtime.

My memory of the next day still brings tears to my eyes. I was woken by my youngest son, tugging at my elbow, saying excitedly, 'Mummy, Cloud Boy chose me to be his friend!' And when I looked out from my bed, there was Jamie, cradling Cloud Boy in his arms and beaming with joy.

This doll then became my son's closest companion, and life at home was transformed. Everywhere that Jamie went, Cloud Boy went with him. When Jamie was given new gumboots, red felt boots were made for Cloud Boy. When Jamie started school, a backpack was sewn for Cloud Boy and a matchbox was filled with raisins for his lunch and put into the backpack. And of course, for the next few years, Cloud Boy slept in Jamie's bed every night. Around the age of nine, Jamie carefully placed him in a basket in his cupboard.

Many years later, when Jamie was studying at university for his Bachelor of Design, he was home visiting me before I left for work in East Africa. He saw me wrapping up Cloud Boy with other toys and books. I was putting them all in a box to be stored away for three years. Jamie was horrified that I could do this to his lifetime friend, and he took Cloud Boy back to Sydney in his backpack. Cloud Boy now lives on Jamie's bed in his flat along with his girlfriend's favourite cuddly toy from her childhood … both waiting for children to come and play with them!

The moment Cloud Boy entered Jamie's life, his desire for the warrior doll disappeared. Jamie's friends would come and join in tea parties with Cloud Boy and wish they had such a friend too. Cloud Boy became part of our family life in so many ways – he even features on several pages in the family photo album. Jamie recently commented that he thought Cloud Boy, together with all the craftwork and puppetry that was associated with the stories from his childhood, has made an important impact on his design work as an adult. He loves and seeks beautiful things, especially natural forms and materials.

i   *When We Were Very Young* and *Now We Are Six* (see reference section for details)

ii   See book by Rudolf Steiner in the reference section

iii   I have since discovered that if these childhood experiences had happened in a country like Iceland they might have been more accepted by the adults. In this northern country of rock and ice, the 'Hidden Folk' (elves, gnomes, trolls and other spirits) apparently enjoy a natural regard. Proof of these little folk being a widespread phenomenon can be found in stories carried by local newspapers – for instance about humans attempting to construct houses or roads on 'elf' rocks and landforms, and suffering inexplicable set-backs. Some of Iceland's most renowned seers of the 'hidden people' have devised 'elf' maps of their principal habitations, and give normal people an insight into the lives and whereabouts of these beings. Describing them as the 'other side' of nature, comparable to light on the trees and the flowers (whose surroundings dictate the form they take), they believe the elves want people to preserve nature. According to such seers, most children have a natural ability to perceive the 'little folk'.

iv   Rather than the awkwardness of using both gender forms, I will alternate between them.

3

Weaving Stories into the Teaching Fabric

As well as being central to my family life, the healing light of stories has interwoven with my professional life – from early childhood education to teacher training, counselling work and parent support programmes, in both Australia and Africa.

In this chapter I describe my journey and struggles as a teacher and counsellor to create stories for diverse behaviours and situations. The examples progress through early years teaching, the lower primary grades, and into my adult counselling work. They have been chosen to illustrate a range of approaches to story making. The full stories relating to each example can be found later in the book. There are also 'tip' boxes, included here to help enthusiastic storywriters. The following section, 'Writing Therapeutic Stories' explores story making and story structure in a more systematic and detailed way.

Poetry leads to story making

After several years devoted to fulltime parenting, both in Africa and Australia, I re-entered the work force by founding a kindergarten on Australia's north-east coast. Story time was the 'heart' of the day, and stories were mostly brought to life through telling, not reading (the subject of 'storytelling' is addressed in more depth at the end of the book). In planning my story programme, I sourced folk tales from all over the world, and slowly experimented with writing simple nature stories for my groups of children. As my kindergarten was in a little town close to a forest, many of my first nature stories were forest tales.

At first my writing started with simple poetry. I never imagined back then that I could actually write a whole story! Writing poetry had been an enjoyable hobby since my teenage years, and a way to express feelings and frustrations. So without any planning, poetry rekindled an imaginative fire in me and quite naturally became my springboard into story making.

One of my poems grew out of a need to keep control of my class on a nature walk. I had decided to take my kindergarten group on their first excursion to the forest close to the school. As we reached the path that led through the trees, the group scattered in every direction, some children even reaching the other side of the forest, right by the main road. With the help of my assistant, I spent the next twenty minutes frantically rounding up the group and then we hastily led them back to school. What I hoped would be a pleasant bushwalk turned into a wild and scary experience for a fledgling teacher!

Before considering any more bushwalks in my kindergarten programme, I visited the forest by myself, desperate for some creative ideas. As I reached the path, I noticed a large tree with what looked like a 'door' at the bottom. This gave me ideas for a poem about a 'Knocking-Door-Tree', and over the following months and years, the poem led to many stories. One of the Knocking-Door-Tree Forest Stories, 'Jaden and the Fairy Eggs', is included later in the book (see page 205).

I know a little secret about a Knocking-Door-Tree,
A Knocking-Door-Tree that waits for you and waits for me.
At the edge of a forest of shimmering green,
With a pathway that leads to where the little folk are seen.

Knock three times, no more, just three,
Then wait together by the Knocking-Door-Tree.
And if together very quietly you wait,
The little folk may come and open up their magic gate!

After that first 'wild' experience, I would gather the class near the tree before any walk through the forest, and recite the poem. This made an enormous difference to the mood of the bushwalk. Without any prompting from me, the children would all delight in taking turns 'knocking' on the door, with the older ones making sure the younger ones didn't knock more than three times! Then I would cup my hand over my ear and say, 'Listen, I can hear the gate opening. Follow me and we shall see what we shall see'. This ensured that I was always the leader and the wild running was channelled into careful walking and watching. We would see lizards, birds, butterflies and dragonflies, and the children were sure they often saw little folk dancing in the sunbeams shining through the trees. In this way we were able to spend much longer times enjoying the forest. Then I was able to deliver the children safely back to the school, often stopping at the park where they could have time to climb and swing and run freely within a safe, fenced area.

The use of poetry and simple rhyme, as well as being a springboard into story making, has since been incorporated in many ways into my story writing. I quickly learnt from telling stories to groups of young children that it was often the repetition and rhyme that kept their concentration. Afterwards the children would take the rhyme into their play in many helpful and healing ways. One example here is the story of 'Benjie and the Turnip' (see page 196). I have seen how its simple rhymes have a powerful effect on children when playing in the garden. Children who may have been tempted to pull up the vegetables and pluck the flowers at random, have been beautifully restrained by this story and have been overheard asking 'Gnome, gnome, good root gnome, may I take your 'turnip' (or 'carrot' or 'flower') home?' I then watch as they bend down to listen to a 'yes' or a 'no'. If necessary, I may whisper from behind, speaking on behalf of the plant, 'Not yet, it's still mine, try again another time!' In a jolly and rhythmical way, this story teaches the deep wisdom of indigenous peoples who have always appreciated their strong connection to the land and its produce. The wisdom is about asking first, and then thanking Mother Earth for her bountiful goodness. Quite a lesson for our snatch-and-grab materialistic age!

STORY TIP
Use poetry as a springboard into story writing. Write your own poems or take a classic poem or nursery rhyme and turn it into a small story. Allow rhyme and repetition to become an integral part of the story.

From the forest to the sea

After years of fundraising and building, my kindergarten finally moved out of rented premises into a permanent home, away from the forest and closer to the beach. Although we continued to pay return visits to the 'knocking-door-tree forest' for school excursions, with the move to the coast the focus of my nature stories slowly changed to sea-side tales.

My inspirations often came from walking on the beach, sitting on the headland looking out to sea or paddling in the rockpools. I am convinced that what the Bushmen People of Southern Africa say is true: 'A story is like the wind, it comes from a far-off place and you feel it'.[i] To get inspiration for a story it so often helps to be out in nature – where you can feel the story winds blowing!

One year, just before Christmas, I was walking along the beach when a tumbleweed came rolling down from the sand-dunes. A little child was running behind trying to catch it. In an instant, I had an idea for a story. The tumbleweed looked so much like a grass star, and reminded me of the rolling and tumbling group of boys in my kindergarten. I had recently seen a grass star used by a friend as an Australian summer Christmas decoration (with gold glitter sprinkled in the centre and hung from the rafters on her verandah). These images swirled in my head, along with the classic rhyme and sequencing pattern of 'The Gingerbread Man' story.

STORY TIP

Use a theme from a classic and well-loved children's story to help construct your own story

---

Finally my 'Grass Star Man' story was born (see page 202), and used that year, and for many years later, as one of the Christmas stories in the kindergarten. In brief, it was about a little old woman who was trying to catch a grass star on the beach. But the grass star didn't want to be caught, he was on his way back up to the sky!

Play, play – no, not I, I'm on my way back up to the sky,

I've no time to play for fun, I belong back up with the sun –
Run, run, run as fast as you can,
You can't catch me – I'm the grass star man!

And he continued rolling along the sand – roly-poly, tumble-bumble, over and over, with the little old woman running after him (soon to be joined by a dog, a crab and some fishermen).

The wild tumbling and restlessness is eventually transformed into stillness and satisfaction, and the little old woman takes the grass star home to hang in her house 'as a Christmas light on Christmas night'.

Interestingly enough, the 'Grass Star Man' story was a real favourite of my rolling, tumbling group of boys. It was the first story of the term that held them in full concentration and stillness, from the first to the last word. This story-time concentration also reached into other daily activities, a small healing in itself.

STORY TIP
Find inspiration in nature. Go walking on a beach or in a forest. Sit quietly in a garden and observe the pulsing life and busy-ness of the natural world.

The patterns, rhythms and metaphors in the natural world can offer unlimited ideas for storymaking. I was once collecting tiny pebbles on the beach, thinking, as I stuffed them into the pocket of my skirt, that I might use these for a puppet show one day. The following week I was driving home and saw by the side of the road an upside-down tree root. It was clean and shiny from the rain, and when turned upright its roots formed a space underneath that looked like a little house. My boys helped me lift it into the boot of the car and deliver it to the kindergarten. These items from nature set my imagination swirling. With the collected nature props, and focusing on the need for a 'sensible sweeping' story for my older children (who had been getting quite wild at cleanup time), my 'Little Straw Broom' puppet show came into being (see page 220).

This broom story has been used with great success and appreciation with all ages of children and adults. I have told it to eight- and nine-year-olds, and afterwards had the class delight in making it into a picture book. I once performed it as a one-person play on stage at an adult storytelling festival. The common consequence of the story is that the listeners start 'itching' to sweep – I have had many parents from my kindergarten ask me 'Why is my child coming home and wanting to know where the broom is?' I have also had both a mother and a father say to me how this story helped them review their share of effort in relation to domestic chores.

> STORY TIP
> Collect props from nature both to inspire your story making and to use with your storytelling – seedpod boats, shells, nuts, acorns, feathers, bamboo and driftwood – the patterns, shapes and textures in the natural world offer unlimited ideas as props for story themes.

A fire story to heal trauma

Sometimes a specific situation seems to dictate a story line. One day at pre-school a normally very settled four-year-old boy arrived like a whirlwind. Matthew proceeded to knock things over and tip things upside-down, and playtime was extremely challenging for all concerned.

His mother, while putting her son's bag into his locker, explained that the previous evening a fire in the home had burnt half their house down. Matthew and his family had escaped to the garden and watched all the bedrooms burn to the ground. His mother had tried to explain to her son that the house was covered by insurance and they would be able to re-build soon, but of course Matthew had been deeply affected by the whole experience. That morning at school, Matthew's behaviour was like the flames of a fire!

Finally it was lunchtime followed by our daily rest, and Matthew fell fast asleep, totally exhausted. While lying down with the children an idea for a story came to me, a story that I thought might help Matthew understand, in a more imaginative way, the traumatic event of the previous evening.

Rabbits were Matthew's favourite animals so I chose a rabbit family for the main characters in the story. My simple story line was about a bushfire that swept quickly across a grassy field and left the baby rabbits sleeping safely deep down in their burrow. After the fire it took several weeks for the green grass to grow again but soon the babies were once again frolicking and jumping around in their grassy playground. My message, through the use of metaphor, was twofold – the rabbit children were safe, and slowly their environment was returned to normal. This story proved to be an example of the powerful effect of using an imaginative rather than a rational explanation for a young child.

I waited until Matthew had woken up, and then gathered the whole group of children for a story time on the veranda, just before the parents arrived. Even though there was no time to 'polish' the story, the whole group loved it, and for the next two weeks they asked to hear it over and over again. The story also had an immediate and remarkable effect on Matthew. When his mother arrived a few minutes later he ran to meet her at the gate and patted her on the arm and said, 'Don't worry Mummy, everything's going to be alright!' She looked at me and said, 'What have you done, Susan?' I suggested that she call me later that night when her children were asleep and I would tell her a story. Which I did! I have included the story later in the book, entitled 'Mother Rabbit and the Bushfire' (see page 230).

STORY TIP
Don't be afraid to try out an idea – a story doesn't always have to be 'in print' and 'polished' to be effective!

A wild pony story

'Restless Red Pony' was written for a four-year-old boy who was exhibiting wild behaviour in a childcare environment. He would run around kicking and hitting other children and found it hard to keep still. He also didn't like being touched, and would lash out at anyone who came near him. The teaching staff felt he needed one-to-one supervision for the safety of the group, and they also started to confiscate his boots so that if he kicked out his bare feet would do less damage to those close to him.

I was called into the childcare centre in an advisory role, and found the boy on the veranda making great protests about having his boots taken off. I sat down and admired the shiny brown boots, and he started to tell me that these were cowboy boots and how one day he wished he could have his own horse. This gave me the idea for the main metaphor in the story that I wrote later that week. The boy loved horses and soaked up the images (see page 199).

The teacher told the story many times, and, following my suggestion, chose to finish each day with a pony game. This game encouraged the children one by one to gallop round the circle then take their place in the centre to be stroked and brushed by all the others – just like restless red pony. The wild boy was one of the first to want to lie down and be brushed. This contact game helped to break the pattern of his aggression.

The story has a general use for kindergarten teachers with groups of boisterous and/or restless children. Of course such behaviour also needs other strategies. With the boy mentioned above, the teachers had to take off his boots to prevent him hurting other children with his wild kicks. A home visit helped understand the problem, and built some consistent approaches between home and school. A copy of the story was also given to the boy's parents to read to him at home.

STORY TIP:
Often we get our best ideas from the children. Listen to their interests, hopes and wishes. Try to incorporate these into your choice of metaphors and journey when writing a story for a specific child or group (refer to the story writing section for more ideas here)

A simple shoe story

In the late 1990s I was working as a field worker for the Centre for Creative Education in Cape Town. This involved visits to the 'Educare' pre-school centres in the townships and squatter camps. My task was to write reports about the trainees, which included some older and more experienced teachers. At one particular school the unspoken feeling with the older woman in charge was that any critical comment I made could affect our friendship, and stir up complex racial issues.

However, there was a glaringly obvious situation that needed attention – fifty pairs of shoes and boots thrown in a pile by the children outside the kindergarten door at rest-time. A teacher then took more than half an hour to sort out the shoes for the children before home time. Instead of making any comment to the head teacher, I made up the following simple story to offer the children (see 'Tembe's Boots' on page 118). The idea came from looking down at my own pair of red boots, which looked like 'friends together'. The head teacher loved the story and continued telling it to the children. From that time on, without any prompting, the older children placed the shoes on the veranda together in beautiful order. Out of pure imitation, the younger ones soon joined in, and the shoe-sorting teacher was able to take a much-needed break instead.

On my next visit to this centre, my first sight was a long line of shoes neatly placed along the veranda. A new and very healthy habit had been established for the children. I have since used this story with many other pre-school and school groups to help establish a shoes-together habit in the first week of the year. It could also have value for families who prefer a 'shoes-off' at the door approach.

STORY TIP
An effective story theme can often be simpler than you think!

Environmental healing tales

An example of a healing story on a universal theme for all age groups is one that I wrote for World Environment Day in 1992. This was then turned into a one-hour musical play by 'Home Grown Productions', Byron Bay, and toured through many primary schools. Entitled 'Garden of Light' (see page 127), it is an example of how drama can strengthen the healing aspect of storytelling.

The play was created in cooperation with the local Seed Saver's Network which provided packet of seeds for the children in the audience to take home and plant in their gardens. The story line had quite a powerful effect on the audience. I watched adults wiping away tears. One class of seven-year-olds, who were meant to be going to the beach after watching the play, insisted that their teacher take them in the bus back to the school so they could start to prepare some gardens and plant their seeds immediately!

The central metaphor for this story is a great golden ball that can shine light into the world only when it is polished each day by the Nature Weaver (using a cloth woven from fresh grasses, flowers and leaves). When King-Didn't-Care comes along and destroys the natural environment, there is nothing left to make a polishing cloth to polish the ball. The ball turns a tarnished grey and the King orders a high stone wall to be built around it to keep it out of sight. When the wall is completed the king starts to turn 'grey' and grows very ill.

The metaphor of the golden ball symbolised for me the universal source of life. Hence when the ball loses its golden shine and the King tries to hide its ugliness, the 'greyness' and imbalance surfaces in him. This loss can never really be hidden or suppressed. Only the innocence and enthusiasm of the children, combined with the wisdom and patience of the Nature Weaver, Mother Earth, could restore the balance.

Many adults saw the play and had different interpretations of the metaphors. The golden ball to some was the divine source or 'God'; to others it was the connector of all things; to others our 'spiritual conscience'. The Nature Weaver was understood by some as a 'God' or 'Goddess', by others as a symbol of the modern environmental movement. These different interpretations emphasise how a story has a life of its own.

Of course, with the young children, it is best not to give or ask for interpretations – this could kill the magic! However, with older primary school and high school ages, the story could be effectively used as a springboard for environmental lessons and debates.

Another example of an environmental healing story is 'Grandmother and the Donkey' (see page 123). Its gentler theme and shorter, simpler journey makes it more suitable for the pre-school and kindergarten ages. Written to encourage litter awareness in Cape Town in 1997, it was toured as a puppet show through kindergartens in the townships. The healing effect of the story on the children was immediate – after each performance, as I and Maria Msbenzi, the other puppeteer, were packing up the show, the children would run up to us with handfuls of litter collected from their school playground. Each day we found that we had to take extra bags and boxes in our car to carry all the garbage.

STORY TIP

Turning a story into a play or puppet show can strengthen the message and healing potential

---

Knitting needles and pocket knives

Even though I have mainly taught in early childhood situations, I have sometimes been called in for relief teaching or for craft teaching at local primary schools. No matter what the subject, telling a story has been my way into the lesson.

One of my most successful experiences was in a series of knitting lessons with 8-year-olds. I had only had one session previous to this with the class, and I found them to be the wildest group of 8-year-olds I had ever met. There were 23 children in the class, 17 were boys, and they were climbing on desks and through the windows when I first walked in.

My plan was to have the children first make their own 'bush' knitting needles – using dowel rods, sharpened at one end with a pencil sharpener, sanded smooth, and a gum-nut glued on the other end. But I was concerned they would start fighting with the knitting needles, or think that knitting was 'un-cool' and not be interested in joining in the lesson.

After much thought (and a sleepless night!) I made up a story about two 'magic sticks' that were found by a boy who was always very bored and up to no good. Entitled 'Jeremy and the Magic Sticks' (see page 162), it was my recounting of the terrible things that this boy did to hurt others that first got the attention of the class. After a series of incidents in the story, a set of 'magic' sticks helped this boy make many amazing things, and whenever he had the sticks with him, with the help of a ball of wool, he was never bored again.

This story captured the imagination of every member of the class. They couldn't wait to make their own 'magic sticks' and, like the boy in the story, knitted amazing things. The knitting lessons for the rest of the term became their favourite time of the week.

My strongest memory of the lessons was the preparation of the knitting needles. The children had to sand their sticks until they were extremely smooth. They had to come out to my desk and rub them against my cheek until I agreed that they felt like velvet. Not once did any of the children try to hurt other children with their precious 'magic' sticks. The story had 'healed' the difficult behaviour and settled the whole class into productive work.

STORY TIP:

Use a story to introduce a lesson (no matter what the subject!). The story will help to create an imaginative connection to the topic and greatly increase the chance that the children will be enthused from the beginning to the end of the lesson.

Another story, 'The Pocket Knife and the Castle' (see page 119), written for seven- to nine-year-olds, was requested by a parent whose son was being irresponsible with tools. The story was used by the parent on the boy's birthday to accompany his special pocket knife present. It made a noticeable difference to how the boy treated his new possession. The story tells about a knife that 'itched' to be used. This was emphasised by the knife having a song of its own. The repetition of the little rhyme helped to create the mood and tension, even for a boy as old as eight.

There was once a young boy who had been given a pocket knife for his birthday. A brand new pocket knife, a gleaming shining pocket knife. A very sharp pocket knife, that itched to be used.

He kept it in his pocket – and there it stayed, itching to be used.

'I am a knife and I love to cut; Open me, use me, then shut me back up'.
The boy was sure he could hear it singing to him sometimes...

I have also successfully used this story in schools and vacation-care programmes to encourage older children to create things with their hands – in wood or clay or soapstone. The knitting needles and pocket-knife stories both show the powerful effect of a story on transforming wild and irresponsible behaviour into productive and settled activity.

STORY TIP:
Incorporate rhymes, riddles and songs into your storytelling. Their repetition helps create the mood and tension in the story. It is often the rhyme that the children remember most, even primary-aged children.

Tales from the story doctor

Another facet of my early childhood work has been parent consultation. I had the privilege of piloting a 'Creative Parent Support' programme for a 'Developing Stronger Families' project funded by the Australian Government. This work involved home visits to families and visits to local schools where I observed parents and teachers struggling with difficult situations. Often the visit was followed up by me writing a story, or encouraging the parent or teacher to write a story, to help or heal difficult behaviour.

In this role with Parent Support I often felt like a 'story doctor'. Over a two-year period, I had many experiences with stories addressing different behaviour challenges in children. Some stories were used by teachers and effected positive change in the school environment, e.g. Restless Red Pony, and A Little Boy went Sailing. Some of the stories were written by and for parents and reached the child in their home environment – e.g. The Ball of Wool, The Magic Stick. Some stories had an influence on the whole family – e.g. Princess Light, The Beautiful Queen. Occasionally a story affected change through touching the parents' imagination – 'Now I get it, I need to give my child more time to be a child' said two different parents after reading about the little brown zebra who was in a hurry to have his stripes turn black. After this feedback, 'Impatient Zebra' became the introduction to my talks on 'Protecting Childhood'.

Other stories had an effect on therapist, parent and child, e.g. 'The Farmer "Just Right"' story helped the family psychologist use an imaginative approach with a five-year-old who climbed into cupboards to go to the toilet. The psychologist then went on to self-publish a little picture book for toileting difficulties with older children. The story helped the mother introduce more routines and consistency into family life, and the child's behaviour was positively affected by the consistency that was now replacing chaos in the home. The child loved the farmer's chant, 'A place for everything and everything in its place'. He was often overheard using this with his toys at tidy-up time. This combination of strategies helped heal the 'out-of-balance' behaviour and the child started to use the toilet again.

These experiences increased my commitment to finding ways to include and encourage the 'light of story' in modern family and school life. The work then extended to running Creative Discipline courses for parents, teachers and therapists. In these courses the participants were helped to use imaginative rhymes, games and stories to meet different discipline challenges. The workshops produced some interesting and successful results, confirming for me and the participants the importance of metaphor and story in child-rearing practices. A selection of the stories from these experiences, both mine and the Creative Discipline workshop contributions, have been included in the story sections of the book.

Writing and sourcing, sifting and sorting

It was the success of all of these experiences that encouraged me to write and collect therapeutic stories and to continue to keep notes documenting their use and effect. These stories and notes have piled up in boxes and drawers, and have slowly been transferred to my trusty laptop. The final outcome is this book.

At this stage, it is probably important to point out that not all my stories have made it into print. Some stories have been scribbled or typed and then put straight into the recycle bin. Others have been put into a file to gather dust. Some of these have been reworked many years later (possibly a message here – *Don't throw any away!*).

There can be many reasons why a story may not 'work', but it is a worthwhile experience to try, and try, and try again. I am convinced that writing dud stories (or 'dories') is an important part of the learning process. Occasionally a story has been so disastrous that after telling it once in my kindergarten, instead of repeating the story for several days (usually a wonderful rhythm for storytelling with young children as they thrive on repetition) I have gone back the next day and told a well-loved folk tale for the rest of the week. Perhaps the story didn't 'work' because it was too long, or perhaps the story journey was too wishy-washy, or too complex? Or perhaps there was too much description and not enough activity?

The next section offers a framework for exploring the above questions, plus other aspects of story structure and many tips for story making.

i   'A Story Like The Wind' by Laurens van der Post (details in reference section)

SECTION TWO

WRITING THERAPEUTIC STORIES

The aim of this section is to share a construction model for story making that has helped me and many workshop participants create healing stories for children. However, before setting off on an exploration of therapeutic story writing, some fundamental questions about 'story' and 'behaviour' need to be addressed.

4

'Story' and 'Behaviour'

What is a story?

I find 'story' as difficult to define as a human or a tree or a rainbow. Is this because it is alive? 'Story', like life, is difficult to define or categorise.

You can look up the definition of 'story' in the dictionary, but you may find, like I did, that it is rather dry:

A piece of narrative, tale of any length told or printed in prose or verse, of actual or fictitious events...

A more 'living' approach is to attempt to describe story in an imaginative or metaphorical way. The following examples show that there can be many different metaphors, and they all work to enrich our understanding of what story is. After reading these, you may find it valuable to think of your own metaphor.

Some metaphors for 'story'

As we saw in Chapter 3, the Bushmen or 'San' people of Southern Africa compare a story to the wind, believing that it comes from a far-away place.

This description captures the heart or 'feeling' connection of a storytelling experience, and seems to say much with few words. Stories are one of the Bushmen's survival tools, influencing key actions in their daily lives, especially the hunt, and teaching about desert animals that will lead them to food and water. The connection of a story to 'the wind' links their imaginary world to their physical world on a daily basis.

The Xhosa women attending my early childhood training in Cape Town compared a nourishing story to a cooking pot full of healthy food. They found this metaphor a wonderful one to use when trying to list the ingredients needed for the 'pot' to write (cook up) a 'nourishing' story for children. They suggested that there could even be a second bowl or pot that contains all the spices that one could add to a story – humour, a riddle, 'magic', a song or rhyme.

Images of 'water', with its many linking metaphors, are a wonderful way to describe the nature of story. Stories are as important to our soul life as water is to our physical well-being – they can rejuvenate and are vital for healthy growth and development; they find their way right into our hearts, into our being, just as water can find a way in through a crack in the wall when nothing else can! Many stories together make a 'well' for life's travellers to dip into and continue on their journey enlivened and refreshed.

Another metaphor for 'story' is 'medicine'. C.P. Estes, in her book *Women who run with the Wolves,* uses story medicine in helping women reconnect with their instinctual selves. Anita Johnston, in her book *Eating in the Light of the Moon,* uses medicinal stories for healing eating disorders. These books are wonderful reading. They draw on the wisdom of myths and folk tales for healing maladies of the soul and body.

Stories as medicine naturally relates strongly to the theme of this book. The therapeutic or healing wisdom of stories has been understood and used throughout human history. Thousands of years of human striving have produced a multiplicity of narratives that often live in many dimensions, with healing messages and meanings that reach from the everyday to the divine.

What is a therapeutic story?

All stories have therapeutic or healing potential. If a story makes people laugh, the laughter can be healing. If a story makes them cry, this can be healing too. Folk and fairy tales, through their universal themes and resolutions, have healing possibilities. They can offer hope and courage to face the trials of life and help the listener find ways to move forward.

David Suzuki, a world-renowned environmentalist, suggests that stories can help in 'healing' our earth by building a spiritual connection to 'place'. If a simple nature story, for example, can help connect children to their local forest, they may be more conscious of protecting it and caring for it when they get older. Through stories a holistic relationship to the environment can be developed and strengthened.

The very experience of listening to a story, no matter what the content, can be 'healing'. Storytelling used on a regular basis in school programmes can help develop and strengthen children's concentration and activate their imaginations. These effects are a healing balm in our modern times when children often spend many hours in passive mode watching TV and DVDs.

But over and above the healing potential of all stories, specific stories can help or heal specific situations. These stories, for the purposes of this book, are described as 'therapeutic'. In line with the definition of healing cited earlier – *restoring to health; bringing into balance; becoming sound or whole* – therapeutic stories can be described as ones that help restore lost equilibrium, or regain a sense of wholeness. When teachers, psychologists, parents, grandparents (and any other adults in a childcaring role) use a healing story with children, the story has the potential to bring the behaviour or situation back towards balance.

What is behaviour?

The word 'behaviour' in relation to children simply means 'the way a child acts'. This can be either positive (co-operative, helpful, sharing, pleasant, reliable, honest, etc.) or negative (aggressive, dishonest, lazy, disrespectful, greedy, irritating, etc.).

Influences on children's behaviour
A child's behaviour may be influenced by many factors:
- Age and stage of development – physical, cognitive, social, emotional
- Individuality (temperament, personality, etc.)
- Cultural background
- Meeting of basic needs (is the child behaving inappropriately because he is hungry, cold, tired, etc.?)

- State of health/well-being
- Family environment
- Daycare, pre-school or school environment
- Presence, or lack of, routines and consistency – in both home and school environments
- Other adults, older children, peers, siblings
- How the child has learnt behaviour in the past – e.g. if screaming loudly, or sulking, always gets the child what he wants, then this can become an entrenched, 'learned' behaviour

All children will display inappropriate or undesirable behaviour at some time. In fact some forms of behaviour considered to be a problem are simply an age-appropriate response to particular stimuli or situations. It is normal for a two-year-old to throw tantrums when limits are enforced. It is normal for a three-year-old sometimes to pocket a toy from daycare to take home – this is not stealing, but an innocent 'borrowing', and may mark the need to create a transition between the child's two realities. It is normal behaviour for a six- or seven-year-old to become a little sneaky, secretive, even dishonest. This doesn't mean that the caregiver has to accept such responses, but it is important that all adults who work with young children have a background understanding of developmental stages and 'norms'. This can be accessed in parenting and educational books on child development and child psychology.[i]

Context and relationships

Most influences on children's behaviour fall into two main categories – context and relationships. Each child exists and develops within an intricate web of environments and networks – family, school, community and global. A child's particular behaviour can rarely be effectively addressed in isolation.

Firstly the context of how, when, where and why certain behaviour occurs are important factors that need to be taken into account. If a child is hungry and/or tired, demanding behaviour is usually predictable and justified. If a child has chronic muscle pains in his legs, and his parents/teachers have not identified this (and the child is not old enough to articulate that he is in pain), then this child may hit out at anyone who comes too close. Consequently he could be incorrectly diagnosed as a child with aggressive tendencies!

I once heard about a four-year-old boy who was behaving in silly and inappropriate ways during 'outside' time at pre-school, particularly when his friends were having fun with mud or water play. On consulting the parents, it was found that this boy had been traumatised six months previously by a mud-flood coming in the back door of the house. Even though the family had recently moved to a new house in the town, the child would not go near mud or water, and would get quite disturbed if he encountered either. The child's father attended one of my therapeutic story workshops and made up a story about a family who lived in a 'bamboo cottage' that always seemed to get full of muddy water when it rained (the story was quite light and humorous). Finally the family packed up and moved to another town and lived in a house with strong walls, many drains and a high fence and were now protected from water coming into their home. Both parents told this story to their son on many nights before bedtime. The boy loved the story and asked for it over and over again. Weeks later it was reported that he was happily playing outside at pre-school and seemed to be delighting in his new discovery of mud, sand and water.

Another example of the influence of 'context' on behaviour was of a boy in my kindergarten who witnessed a fire burn down half his house. I described this in Chapter 3.

Secondly, the child's relationship to others in the group and/ or the family can have an influence on behaviour. Has the child recently joined the class or the family recently moved to a new area? There is often a behaviour pattern that children can bring to new relationships – a more extrovert child may enter a new peer-group and find her place through 'show-off' behaviour, whereas a shyer child may behave in a needy/clinging way. This requires under- standing from the teacher/parents and some nurturing attention to help the child find her way in the first few weeks or months. Some time is important here for allowing the behaviour to 'settle down' or return to 'normal'. This doesn't mean teachers/parents ignore possible challenging behaviour. They need to be continually observant and alert to the social dynamics in children's groups. They especially need to be aware of any signs of bullying. An example of how a teacher dealt with bullying with an eight-year-old girl who recently joined the class can be found in 'Red Truck Story' (see page 191). Kim Payne's work on social inclusion and bullying is recommended reading (see website in reference section).

Another example of the effect of relationships on behaviour is when the child is one of the youngest in the family. Early childhood teachers often observe that the younger children in a family bring to school the behaviour they have experienced from their older siblings – teasing, bullying, bad language, etc. Although stories can have the potential to help here, they may need to be supplemented by a home visit and some strategies for the whole family.

Thirdly, the adult's relationship to the child, and to the situation, can impact on what may be termed 'challenging behaviour'. The 'Baby Bear Koala' story (see page 249) was written for a kindergarten mother who was distressed that her four-year-old child was behaving 'badly' as he didn't want to part from her each day. When the story helped clarify that it was actually the mother who didn't want to part from her child, she realised that the accusation of her child behaving 'badly' was incorrect. The reality of this situation was that the mother had not faced her own fears from being left as a child. She was also feeling guilty for working full-time when the boy was younger and constantly leaving him with a babysitter. The healing story helped bring clarity to her thoughts and a more healthy balance to her relationship with her son. She kept him at home for another year and then he happily started school at age five. Sometimes it is the parent or teacher's behaviour that needs to be addressed!

Other adult/family influences can come from recently separated or remarried parents, resulting in split families and/or newly added stepchildren. In one situation a home visit revealed that the three children (one of them a step-child) were constantly fighting and screaming to get the mother's attention. The mother was in an extremely depressed state over, in her words, her 'lack of worth as a human being'. The children's difficult behaviour had a direct connection with their depressed and stressed mother. I wrote a story for the mother to help her rediscover her inner beauty (see 'The Beautiful Queen', page 165). Not only did the story help the mother feel better about herself, but after reading it many times she decided to share it with her children aged 13, 9 and 5 years. They wanted to hear it again and again. The story was only one strategy on a long path of family therapy, but it helped the family start a bedtime story ritual. The mother reported that at last there was one time in the day when the family felt back in 'balance'.

Evaluating adult influence on children's behaviour

It is important to continually evaluate your approach to care-giving to make sure that you are not contributing to the difficult behaviour – e.g. do your expectations match the child's age and stage of development? Does the school programme meet the child's needs? Are your daily activities organised and prepared? It is also important to check if you are working with strategies that help promote positive behaviour.

The following list may help you (and other parents/teachers/carers in the child's environment) with this evaluation:

• Do you model positive behaviour?
• Do you model positive and respectful language?
• Do you model and teach social skills?
• Do you set clear, fair and consistent limits?
• Do you notice and encourage desirable behaviour?
• Do you re-direct and distract children's negative behaviours where possible (a 'nip in the bud' approach)?
• Do you ignore (or 'feed') attention–seeking behaviour?
• Do you give 'mixed-messages' in dealing with inappropriate behaviour – i.e. say one thing but do another? For example, saying to a child: 'If you continue whingeing, we won't go to the park' while putting the child's walking shoes on in readiness for going there.
• Do you have quality 'time' for/with each child in your care?
• Is your child's day over-scheduled, not allowing for enough free play (down-time)?

Identifying 'challenging' behaviour

Even with the above strategies in place, a child may display behaviour that requires a more considered and individual approach. Termed a 'difficult' or 'problem' or 'challenging' behaviour, it is often more than a short-term annoyance or disturbance. In our care-giving role we usually 'know' if a child is exhibiting challenging behaviour because dealing with it can take up a large amount of the carer's time and emotional energy!

On a more formal level, child psychologists offer extensive descriptions of 'challenging' or difficult behaviour. For the purposes of this book, these have been condensed into the following points.

Challenging or difficult behaviour may be:

- Behaviour that disrupts, harms, or infringes unfairly on the rights of others
- Behaviour that harms the environment or other living things
- Behaviour that presents a clear risk of harm to the child
- Typical behaviour that occurs too often or beyond the age where we would expect a child to learn more appropriate options
- Behaviour that interferes with the child's ability to learn and process information, or prevents the child from using already learned skills
- Behaviour that interferes with the child's ability to interact
- Appropriate behaviour at the wrong time or place (e.g. throwing balls inside the house; loud singing or laughing in the school library)
- Behaviour that is consistently a problem and seen as such by more than one person

---

Challenging behaviour can be further classified as a 'disorder' (e.g. Attention Deficit Hyperactivity Disorder, commonly known as 'ADHD') if a pattern of problems display relative severity, exist in multiple settings, continue over an extended period of time, and interfere with 'normal development'. Children with suspected behaviour disorders should be referred to a team of specialists for diagnosis. To gain a thorough picture, the child's teacher and all relevant care-givers should, where possible, be included in the discussion and diagnostic process.

Describing specific challenging behaviour

Behavioural descriptions need to be clear and precise. General labels like 'timid', 'fearful', 'destructive' or 'uncooperative' make it difficult to understand what it is that needs changing and what the desirable change could be. Most importantly, when we come to story-making, specific descriptions help in choosing metaphors to suit specific behaviours. It can be a helpful exercise to list the following:

- Who is doing the behaviour (and, if applicable, who else is involved)?
- What is the behaviour?
- When does the behaviour occur?
- Where does it occur?
- How does the behaviour manifest?

The following tables (see pages 52-55) have been compiled with examples of challenging and desirable behaviour – both at home and at daycare/school.

Labels and categories

When contemplating a story to address challenging behaviour, it should not be a question of 'bad' behaviour made 'good' through a story, or 'naughty' children made into 'good' children. It is about trying to bring the behaviour or situation back into wholeness or balance. My strong advice to you in playing midwife to this process is to beware of labelling! It is unhealthy practice for children to be labelled, and yet it can happen so easily, and so often with negative results. I have known a child who was mistakenly labelled as 'dishonest' by the teachers in a school and over time he 'grew' into this label. When interviewed by the school counsellor several years later he revealed the following thoughts: 'If I am going to be accused for every theft that happens in the classroom, then I might as well get the benefits of spending the money'.

For an easy reference to stories for commonly identified behaviours, I have found it necessary in this book to use general categories like 'greedy', 'lazy', 'shy', 'restless' in the story sections. These categories could mistakenly be used to describe or label a child.

This is not my intention. The categories could also be read as putting the behaviour problem 'inside' the child, rather than as part of a whole context and relationship. Again, this is not my intention. A description of a particular behaviour should relate to the behaviour only, and should never be confused with the child herself.

We also need to keep in mind that our judgement of whether behaviour is 'good' or 'bad', 'appropriate' or 'inappropriate' can be very subjective. It is influenced by our own beliefs, attitudes, cultural background, past experiences (including our own upbringing), combined with our individual relationship with and understanding of the child and the situation. Sharing our experiences with other parents/teachers / counsellors can help give more objectivity.

Imbalance to balance

An intention to transform or 'heal' challenging behaviour should be seen on a continuum of bringing things back into balance (for example, 'uncaring' to 'more caring'; untidy to tidier; restless to settled; dishonest to honest), not changing a 'bad' child into a 'good' child.

If a four-year-old child is exhibiting demanding and whingeing behaviour – and the family has just moved house or a new baby has arrived – a story to help the demanding child adjust to the new situation could help restore balance in family life (see 'Anything New', page 210).

If five-year-old children are in the habit of throwing their toys around the classroom, an imaginative story line that brings the toys to life can restore respectful and caring balance. The story could build the picture of a doll enjoying being rocked and fed (not thrown), of a little pot and spoon loving to help cook dinner for the doll (not thrown), a car enjoying taking the doll for a ride (not thrown)… But what about the outside toys? A ball that loves to be taken out and thrown up in the air to reach as high as the sky. At the end of play the ball is brought back inside and tucked back into its box to rest next to the doll and other toys. A little rhyme for each toy could be helpful for the adult to use during playtime:

I'm a little doll (car, etc) and it's very well known,
I love to be rocked (pushed along, etc) but never thrown!

Describing 'challenging' behaviour

WHO	WHAT	WHEN	WHERE	HOW
1) Girl – 5 yrs	Fearful of being alone in any room of the house	Day and night	At home	Clings to mother or father – wants someone to be with her whenever she goes to different rooms – e.g. to the toilet / her bedroom
2) Boy – 8 yrs	Irresponsible use of knives	When left alone	At home	Uses sharp knife to cut into furniture, trees, pillows, etc
3) Boy – 4½ yrs	Continual whingeing (whining) to teacher	Inside and outside playtime	At school	Stays close to teacher, complains about having no friends, whinges (whines) about daycare being boring
4) Whole class – 6 yrs	Lack of co-operation at clean-up time	After morning tea and lunch	At school	Children try to run around or hide instead of helping sweep floor, wipe tables, etc

Describing a 'desirable' behaviour

WHO	WHAT	WHEN	WHERE	HOW
1) Girl – 5 yrs	Confident to explore new spaces and be on her own	Day time	At home	Child gains confidence in venturing into and being able to stay by herself in new sections of the house, in daylight hours (child too young to be expected to be confident in the dark)
2) Boy – 8 yrs	Responsible and constructive use of knives and other sharp tools	When left alone	At home	Uses knife and chisels for carving wooden shapes Uses knife in cooking – to chop vegetables, fruit, etc
3) Boy – 4½ yrs	Stops complaining – gets involved in play	Inside and outside playtime	At school	Stops clinging to teacher – gets involved with other children and begins to participate in and enjoy the daily program
4) Whole class – 6 yrs	Co-operation at tidy-up time	After mealtimes	At school	Children enjoy sweeping and cleaning; children co-operate and act sensibly at cleaning up time

Using the medium of story to transform 'challenging' to 'desirable' behaviour

(Note: the framework for writing such stories is explored in the following chapter)

WHO	WHAT	STORY	OUTCOME
1) Girl – 5 yrs	Fearful of being alone in any room of the house	Story about a 'star girl' who comes down from the sky and into a child's bedroom at night through the window. 'Star Girl' becomes the child's special friend	Mother made a 'star doll' as a prop for the story and a star necklace to hang on a hook in the kitchen – her daughter started to wear this. With it hanging around her neck she started to go to the toilet on her own and also to venture into other parts of the house.
2) Boy – 8 yrs	Irresponsible use of knives	Story describes many destructive uses of a pocket knife and its repetitive consequences. This is followed by a dream and the carving of a wooden castle (See 'The Pocket Knife and the Castle' page 119)	Boy experiences the joy of creating something beautiful by carving wood. Boy is motivated to use his pocket knife to construct rather than destroy or damage things.

3) Boy – 4½ yrs	Continual whingeing (whining)	Story about a young whale so busy whingeing he loses his way and gets caught in a shallow lagoon; he is finally rescued by his use of whale song. (See 'Whingeing Whale', page 100)	Teacher uses rhyme and song from story to deal with clinging behaviour in a light way. Child's whingeing replaced by more constructive uses of voice – he starts to copy the rhyme and song. Child slowly detaches from teacher and gets involved in play activities.
4) Whole class – 6 yrs	Lack of co-operation at tidy-up time	Story about three little men who take turns using the broom – one couldn't be bothered, one is too fast and wild, one is careful and committed to the task. (See 'Little Straw Broom', page 220)	Teacher presents puppet show of story. Children act out story with different coloured hats and take this activity into their play and into tidy-up time – 'gold hat' behaviour becomes enjoyable and is encouraged by the teacher and peer-group.

If six-year-olds are continually dropping their lunch scraps and papers into the garden, this littering behaviour could be brought back into balance by the teacher telling and dramatising the 'Grandmother and the Donkey' story (see page 123). The metaphor of caring for 'nature's child', with ways of helping nature's child to be beautiful rather than ugly, can make a deep impact on children. This can help transform their behaviour through their own motivation to make a difference.

If an eight-year-old is found continually stealing, a story that moves, in great detail, through the stealing behaviour and its consequences, can help give the child a more balanced and engaged understanding (see 'Dishonest Dingo', page 110).

The tapestry of discipline

The main aim of this book is to help you to use healing stories to meet challenging behaviour in a subtle but effective way. In this chapter, various strategies have been described to help you understand and identify different kinds of behaviour. In the next chapter I offer a framework to help you find metaphors and construct stories to address a wide range of behaviours and situations.

As stated earlier, storytelling is just one of many possible approaches and strategies in addressing challenging behaviour, and cannot fix all problems. To thoroughly address the bigger picture requires a study of the complex 'tapestry' of discipline. Stories have the potential to be light-filled threads in this tapestry. But if the foundation threads in the weaving are not strong, the fabric can fall apart. Working with healing stories without any 'foundation' could leave story threads hanging in mid-air and very little to show for the creative effort.

This weaving metaphor can be helpful in finding a comprehensive approach to behaviour management with young children. It can provide many useful strategies for challenging behaviours. The strong warp threads include rhythm, routine and consistency, acceptance, respect, setting realistic limits, preparation and organisation, and many other ways and means to help promote positive behaviour (see previous list). The creative weft threads are also numerous. As well as the imaginative thread of storytelling, the discipline tapestry can be coloured and enriched through humour, games, songs, rhymes, family rituals, festivals and community events.

The complex tapestry of discipline requires a separate book (my next project?) devoted to exploring its rich and varied threads. This book however, must confine itself to the single, illumined strand of healing stories.

i   For instance: Rahima Baldwin Dancy, *You Are Your Child's First Teacher* (see reference section)

5

A Construction Model for Story Writing

As will be clear by now, my construction model for writing a therapeutic (healing) story works with a three-part framework of 'Metaphor', 'Journey' and 'Resolution'. To help you as a writer, I now want to identify and discuss these separately, even though you will find they merge intricately to create the finished story.

The framework put forward here is only one possible approach. Please do not see it as the only way to write stories. Use it as a starting point for story making. It may also help you with analysing existing stories, which in the long run can help with the creation of new ones.

First you need to be clear about what you are trying to achieve. In writing a healing story it helps to carefully select therapeutic metaphors and to construct a journey or quest to meet the need of the situation *and* the age of the children. The story should not try to moralise or induce guilt – this cannot be stressed enough! The objective is simply to reflect what is happening and, through the story 'metaphors' and 'journey', provide an acceptable means of dealing with the behaviour and/or a realistic resolution. A healing tale should, as much as possible, leave the listener free to come to her own conclusion – in this way the 'power of story' is left to do its work, as Ben Okri suggests, 'in silence, invisibly'.

Metaphor

The use of metaphor[i] is a vital ingredient in therapeutic story making. Metaphors help build the imaginative connection for the listener. An integral part of the story journey, they often play both the negative roles (the obstacles, tempters and temptations that pull the behaviour or situation out of balance) and the positive roles (the helpers or guides that lead the behaviour/situation back to wholeness or equilibrium). The table of 'Metaphors in story making' below gives some examples of these, but first it may help to look at one example.

Try to picture the following: a story is written for a child who is pinching other children, but the story contains no imaginative metaphor – in other words it is directly about a child who always pinches other children, learning to stop when the other children refuse to be her friend. If such a story is told in class, because it lacks metaphors to help 'lift' the listeners into their imaginations, the group will quite possibly try to work out who the story is about, and suddenly the teacher might be interrupted by someone calling out, 'Rebecca does the same, she pinches everyone!'

Let us now take the same example and build a story with metaphor. Starting first with 'simile' can be a helpful inroad to story making. 'A pinching child is like a nipping crab'. Then drop the 'as if' and 'is like' and our story can begin.

There was once a little crab who was not very popular. His friends were tired of him always being in a cranky mood and using his claws to nip and hurt them …

Now, into the story come some of the 'obstacle' metaphors – Octopus, Starfish, and Seagull. They are the upset friends who plot some unpleasant punishments for Crab. Next, Turtle enters as the wise helper. One more 'helping' metaphor along the story journey is the seaweed mittens that keep Crab's nippers warm and cosy. The resolution is Crab's 'self-progress' towards keeping his nippers under control – eventually the mittens fall apart, the waves wash them out to sea, and Crab is able to play with his friends without hurting them.

This story about 'Cranky Crab' (see page 159) has been used successfully by a therapist and a teacher for pinching behaviour. After the story was first told in class a 'pinched' child asked the teacher to bring some gloves for the pincher. The pincher happily accepted wearing the gloves. The story had presented this idea in a positive light, and not as a punishment.

The table below (see pages 60-61) lists metaphors used in some of the therapeutic stories in this book. It is a guide only – the imaginative qualities of metaphor make them difficult to sort and categorise. You will notice that in one example, 'The Brownies Story', one of the 'obstacles' is also one of the 'guides' – the riddle is an obstacle, but once solved by the boy it becomes a guide towards his new task of becoming a helping Brownie. In the story of 'Tembe's Boots' there are no obstacles, only a slight change when it comes to rest-time and the boots need to wait outside the room. In this story the journey is simply a repetition of the boots as 'friends together'.

As an exercise in understanding the use of metaphor in story making, I suggest you read some other stories from the book, then fill in the empty lines in the table, identifying the obstacles and the helpers. (But you may also find a story that doesn't have metaphors that fit either of these categories!)

Clues for choosing metaphors

When writing a story to address specific behaviour, clues for metaphors for the main character can sometimes come from finding a corresponding animal, bird, insect or object with a similar behaviour – e.g. pinching or nipping crab (a lamb or a dove would not work as a metaphor for pinching!); pesky pelican; restless pony; scratching cat; noisy gnome.

When writing a story for a specific child, metaphors can also be found by using the child's favourite animal or toy, or taking clues from his surrounding environment. Does the child have a passion for dogs, for horses, or for the sea and sailing boats? Does he live by a river, in a forest or in a high-rise block in a city? If in the country or city, what sights and/or daily experiences does the child have on his way to school, in the local forest or on the beach?

Metaphors in story making

Story	Obstacles, tempters, temptations	Helpers, guides
Born to be King (page 230)	The castle walls; the broken bones; the dark room	The wise woman; the mirror; the sunlight; the prince's golden crown; 'born to be king'
Grandmother and the Donkey (page 123)	Move from country to town; people's loss of connection to nature; litter in streets	Grandmother; Nature's Child; donkey; children
Pesky Pelican (page 143)	Always wanting more; food easily available	Advice from the pelican parents; the kind fisherman; remembering what 'pelicans' should really do!
Greedy Possum (page 131)	Bower bird, sparkling 'human' treasures, hollow log to withdraw into; pouch to hold 'things'	Nature's beauty, mother, dewdrop, pouch to hold baby possum
Dishonest Dingo (page 110)	Smallest dingo in litter; red dust; hunger; cave of bones	Cleansing rain; dingo's own conscience

Garden of Light (page 127)	King-didn't-care; treasure mines and treasure castles; high stone wall; grey tarnished ball	Nature Weaver; nature cloth; shining golden ball; children
Whingeing Whale (page 100)	Losing connection with group, reef, shallow water, tide going out	Memory of whale song, whale pod, large wave
The Brownies (page 13)	Cranky father; journey through dark forest; owl and riddle	Grandmother; owl and riddle; boy's realisation of his helping task
Tembe's Boots (page 118)		Little red boots; repetition of 'friends together'

When writing a story for a whole group or class of children, then clues for metaphors may be found from a theme in the curriculum or from the local school environment. There might be a mixture of noisy birds and soft singing birds in the school garden, and a very noisy child in the classroom. This could lead to a story with the theme of listening to others. Perhaps there is inappropriate spitting behaviour in the group. The teacher could connect this with the recent purchase of a new garden hose for the school. In the story, which can be delightfully humorous, the hose could start squirting everything – even a neighbour standing on the other side of the fence, or the secretary working in the office. Finally the hose has to be turned off at the tap and packed away until it realises that there are some things that shouldn't be squirted!

When looking for clues for metaphors, there are no hard and fast rules – stories don't fit comfortably with 'rules'! Sometimes humour can work very well – for example, for a story about stealing, the metaphor of 'sticky fingers' (and a character of the same name) could lead to all kinds of bizarre adventures, where everything touched by the thief gets stuck to him. Sometimes a story may catch the interest of a child because the metaphors are so 'foreign'. Choosing a story for thumb-sucking about a monkey who is always sucking its fingers and toes (and therefore misses out on eating the ripest and sweetest fruits) could work very well for a child who lives in a cold northern country and has never even seen a monkey.

You need to exercise lateral thinking in your choice of metaphors. A colleague once wrote a story for a child whose mother had gone away without any warning and nobody knew when she would return. Even if this child had had a favourite animal, to choose a mother animal for this story would have been difficult. Mothers in the animal kingdom rarely leave their children alone. Instead, this colleague chose to use the moon (mother) and the stars (children) as her metaphors. In her story, called 'Mother Moon' (see page 248), she put the emphasis on the star children in the night sky having to polish their star clothes so they could shine brightly until mother moon returned. Apparently this story helped the relatives as well as the child – they all had to find ways to be stronger until mother returned. The story resolution was careful not to promise any return. Fortunately, however, the mother came back five months later.

Metaphors or story seeds

Metaphors are not just used within stories. They have a power when used on their own that is sometimes so obvious it can be overlooked. Metaphors or 'story seeds' can be wonderful tools for helping behaviour change (examples of the 'magic sash' and the 'waterfall' have already been described in the first chapter).

When my eldest son was five years old he was due for his first dentist appointment. I was quite nervous, as the visit to the dental surgery brought up tense memories from my own childhood. For Kieren however, it was very exciting. He climbed up into the great chair, opened his mouth wide with anticipation and was examined. The dentist, an old Indian man, then told Kieren that one of his teeth was in need of a silver star to make it strong. He explained that it would hurt a little as he put the star inside, but the star would live there for a long time and take care of his weak tooth. 'Would this be ok?' he asked. Kieren nodded an enthusiastic YES, and the procedure began.

This was an interesting lesson for me in the power of metaphor – in this case, a 'silver star' – in making a positive difference to Kieren's acceptance of having a filling put into his tooth. Kieren quite happily returned to the dentist a year later – there was no difficult behaviour to deal with to get him there. My only difficulty with the whole experience was that my second son was upset that he didn't get a star as well! I had to convince him that it was best to have your own teeth naturally strong and the stars were only used to strengthen them.

It is through the use of metaphor or 'story seeds' that poets, writers and politicians can often deliver such potent messages. Metaphors are also part of our everyday life, for instance when we describe character traits ('quiet as a lamb', 'slippery as an eel') and in emphasising various predicaments ('opening a can of worms', 'taking the bull by the horns', 'setting the cat amongst the pigeons'). At the weekly teachers' meeting a colleague might say something like: 'We should leave no stone unturned until this problem is solved'. This kind of language, with a pictorial element, often makes greater impact. Metaphor is ubiquitous in language, though it can easily also become cliché through over-use, thus losing its original, striking power. Poets and creative storytellers also revive and refresh language itself, giving it a new charge and lease of life.

I encourage you to work more consciously with metaphor with your children. Choose a child's behaviour that you are finding difficult at the moment. A simple example: tidying up the toys. How could a visual image or metaphor make a difference to the situation? Firstly think of something that is a tidy and methodical character: An animal? An insect? A little elf? When you have made your choice, try to create a little rhyme for your child to use at tidy-up time – e.g. *As tidy as a little elf, putting things back on the shelf* ... This could then be extended into a short story, with one or more 'obstacle' metaphors to cause untidiness then a 'helping' metaphor (the one from your rhyme) to bring 'tidiness' back into the room or house.

Journey

The journey is the structural part of the therapeutic story construction. An eventful journey is a way to build the 'tension' as the story evolves, and can lead the plot into and through the behaviour 'imbalance' and out again to a wholesome resolution. The use of 'obstacle' and 'helping' metaphors are intricately connected with the journey. The tension or conflict in the journey is usually built up through the involvement of the 'obstacle' metaphors, and the resolution is achieved through the 'helping' metaphors.

For a 3-4 year-old, the 'journey' can be as simple as using repetition of the same experience, or the repetition of a song or rhyme throughout the story. In 'The Snail and the Pumpkin' (see page 201), the snail's song is repeated many times as she travels up and over the pumpkin mountain: *'Slowly, slowly, oh so slow, this is how a snail must go'.* In 'The Little Straw Broom' (see page 220), written to enthuse willing helpers, the repetition of the 'crumbs' poem builds the journey tension. After the children have heard this three times, they are thirsting for a positive solution, for the crumbs to be swept up.

Another way of building tension is by using repetition combined with a sequence of additional characters (often referred to as 'cumulative' stories). The repetition becomes the key structural device in the story by developing the action through a single extending image. The well known tale of the 'The Enormous Turnip' is an excellent example here – a little boy tries to pull up the turnip, then calls mother, who calls grandfather, who calls rabbit; rabbit calls mouse; and finally mouse calls caterpillar. There are countless versions of this story from cultures around the world. Without the build-up of characters, the story would simply be a recounting of a quite insignificant incident – 'A boy went into the garden and pulled up his turnip'.

In a story for an older child, the story 'journey' usually needs to be more involved, with a quest of some kind and several turnings or tasks along the road. In the 'Brownies Story' (see Chapter 2), the twists and turns of the journey lead the listener deep into the story theme. If Grandma had simply told the boy that he is meant to be the helping brownie, it is unlikely that the child would have listened. Instead the story journey takes the boy into the forest to visit the owl, then back to the lake in the moonlight to solve a riddle.

Examples of more complex plots can be found in many of the well-known fairytales such as 'Cinderella' or 'Snow White'. Some examples in this book include 'The Invisible Hunter' and 'Garden of Light'.

To really get a feel of the themes, tension and journey in more complex stories, my advice is to read many children's stories. Try to borrow or buy collections of folktales from many different cultures. There are also internet sites where you can find a wonderful variety of stories (see Bibliography and references).

Resolution

The resolution in a therapeutic story is the restoration of harmony or balance in a situation or behaviour that has been disruptive or out of balance. It is important that the resolution is positive and forward-looking, and not guilt-inducing. For example, in the 'Cranky Crab' story, the pinching behaviour is out of balance and unacceptable to the crab's friends. Through the help of the turtle, the seaweed mittens, and Crab's own efforts, the behaviour is restored to balance. The little crab is not made to feel guilty about his behaviour. Instead the story journey leads naturally to a self-determined resolution. In the 'Bored Baboon' story, (see page 98), the family's efforts to encourage the child to go out and play amount to nothing. Yet the young baboon's lack of interest in playing is clearly out of balance – can you imagine a little baboon just wanting to sit and do nothing? Through the journey of being trapped in the hunter's cage, the out-of-balance experience is taken to the extreme and then resolved by the baboon being rescued and set free to run and jump and play. What a relief for him and the listener!

Even though the resolution comes at the end of the story, it is usually helpful when planning to think about this before anything else. If the resolution is not clear, then it is difficult to know what to work towards with your metaphors and journey.

Different behaviours and situations seem to require different approaches. Some are quite straightforward – for example, in a story for a child who is continually whingeing or whining, the obvious resolution is to have the whingeing replaced by more constructive uses of a voice. In the story of 'Whingeing Whale' (see page 100), the baby whale ends up learning to use his voice to make a beautiful whale song.

A more complex approach is presented in the story of 'Dishonest Dingo' (see page 110). The story leads the listener through sequences of stealing, goes deep into the 'cave of bones', and ends with the cleansing rain unveiling the dishonest mask. The resolution here is that dishonest behaviour changes to honest behaviour through the conscience of the main character, not through any kind of externally imposed punishment.

A less obvious resolution occurs in a story for a child with separated parents. This needs some careful thought – the story should not offer more than what may happen in real life – i.e. don't suggest that the parents might get back together! To help plan the resolution, you may need to make some enquiries. Do the parents communicate and share time with the child? Has one parent disappeared altogether from the family scene? There could also be a chance in such a story for the parents to hear a message and change their behaviour – learning about consistency, for example, and keeping their focus on the child's needs. Perhaps the story could be about two trees growing in different gardens, spreading their shade over a child who plays in both places. The child could move from one garden to the other through a special gate that opens with rhythmical timing. Perhaps the gate opens and closes with a special song? A parent could use this song while driving the child to spend time with the other parent, thus helping to minimise the anxiety that often comes at such times. The story could also include a metaphor of strong sunlight filtering through the trees and giving light to each garden at different times. Perhaps the trees can even have a few branches that reach across the fence and weave amongst each other. Or if this is too 'close', the trees could be in opposite corners of each garden, with the special gate the only link between the two. Working out these different resolutions can be a healing balm for the parents and the therapist/teacher, as well as for the child.

For a child who is terminally ill, it would be inappropriate to make up stories where the sick get better and live happily ever after. The story maker has a serious responsibility to try to capture the bigger picture, with the resolution taking the listener to a place higher, or different, than the earthly one. Parents writing for their own children would most likely work from their own religious and/or philosophical beliefs. Teachers or therapists writing a story need to take the family's beliefs into account. See the stories 'Silky Wriggly' (page 232), 'Stream, Desert, Wind' (page 235) and 'Shimmer Wing' (page 240) for three different examples.

Analysing therapeutic stories

The following tables (see pages 68-73) should be helpful for analysing existing stories, following the model of metaphor, journey, resolution. These analysis exercises may give some clarity to the model and help with new story constructions. Table One lists some examples of stories for general sorts of behaviour. Table Two lists some examples of stories written for specific situations. To get the most from these, I suggest you start with each table and go down the columns one story at a time. First read the story, then come back and fill in the empty columns.

At the back of the book, completed tables are included for Table One and Table Two. However, there are no right or wrong answers – this is only intended as a guide. You may find metaphors or resolutions in a particular story that other readers may not connect with, or perceive. Table Three is empty and is included for photocopying for your own use, or for group use, when brainstorming ideas for new stories.

Table One: ANALYSING THERAPEUTIC STORIES – General types of behaviour

STORY	METAPHOR(S)	JOURNEY	RESOLUTION
Tembe's Boots (page 118)	• Little red boots • 'Friends together'	• A description (with much repetition) of the daily adventures of a pair of boots	• Boots taken off feet and put carefully together at rest-time, not thrown in a messy pile
The Grandmother and the Donkey (page 123)			
Little Straw Broom (page 220)			

Restless Red Pony (page 199)	Whingeing (Whining) Whale (page 100)	Impatient Zebra (page 146)

Table Two: ANALYSING THERAPEUTIC STORIES – Specific Situations

STORY	METAPHOR(S)	JOURNEY	RESOLUTION
Baby Bear Koala (page 249)	• Tree (world) • Hungry growing baby • Tired mother • Juicy leaves • Higher branches	• Mother and baby in tree, mother falls asleep, hungry baby climbs by himself to reach juicy leaves	• Young koala becomes strong enough and brave enough to leave mother and venture into the world by himself
Cranky Crab (page 159)			
The Pocket Knife and the Castle (page 119)			

Born to be King (page 230)	Cloud Boy Story (page 22)	The Towel Story (page 192)

Table Three: CONSTRUCTING THERAPEUTIC STORIES

STORY	METAPHOR(S)	JOURNEY	RESOLUTION

Working out of a 'helping' intention

One of my storytelling students in Nairobi worked at the SOS Children's Village. Towards the end of the training module, she asked me for a story to help with a newly arrived child called Sylvia. Sylvia had recently been orphaned at the age of five after her whole family was killed in a raid on her village.

My first reaction to this request was to say 'No, sorry, I can't possibly do this'. I then asked the student how she thought a story could make any difference to such a horrendous experience in a young child's life. The student pleaded, 'Perhaps a story could help, even if not heal?'

Once back in Australia I worked on a simple story with this aim – hoping to help the situation (see 'A Doll for Sylvia', page 239). Emailed back to Kenya, it was told to Sylvia by her teacher, who later reported on her improved play and interaction with others. The morning after hearing the story Sylvia woke up to find a doll in her bed, dressed in clothes embroidered with silver and gold threads. The doll became Sylvia's special friend.

This was a humbling experience, one that led me to realise that some stories may simply help a little, even where no resolution is possible … and what a bonus if they can! It taught me that the story maker should always work out of this 'helping' intention, with the occasional blessing that a story may indeed 'heal'. Even though this book is about 'healing' stories, I believe it is important to keep this 'helping' intention close to your heart, and be cautious of excessive expectations.

The value of props

The above example of 'A Doll for Sylvia' was given extra strength by the use of a 'prop'. Occasionally a therapeutic story lends itself to this strategy. Adding props to a story does not mean one needs to buy something from a toyshop. There is magic and meaning in the use of a simple homemade item … a crown for a prince made from finger-knitted yellow wool; a stitched felt hat for a helping elf or brownie; a magic leather ring or painted wooden shield as 'protection' for a bullied child.

A therapist used a story strengthened by a prop to help a five-year-old child who was suffering from nightmares and afraid to go into any room in the house without a parent, even in the daytime. The story was about a 'star girl' who came into the child's bedroom at night through the window and became a special friend. The mother made a 'star doll' as a prop for the story and the doll was hung inside her child's bedroom window. At the therapist's suggestion the mother also made a simple star necklace to hang on a hook in the kitchen – she encouraged her daughter to wear this and explore other parts of the house. With the star hanging around her neck the little girl could start going to the toilet on her own, and also into other parts of the house.

A mother from a Creative Discipline course had a successful 'prop' experience with her seven-year-old girl who had recently started to complain about going to school. The mother was travelling as part of her new job and her daughter had become unsettled because she was frequently away, even though the father was at home. The mother made up a story about a little wind fairy that could take messages over the mountains and through the forests, backwards and forwards between friends. Every time the mother returned home she would add adventures to this story. For a prop she sewed a simple little felt doll with white wings. Her daughter started to take it to school – it was small enough to fit inside her pocket – and she would whisper messages to it throughout the day. The prop gave her the security she needed to be at school when her mother was away.

Two parents were having a difficult time with their five-year-old boy not wanting to sleep in his bed in his own room. This family had a new baby, and getting a reasonable amount of sleep each night was a high priority for both parents. Having the five-year-old in their bed as well as the new baby was putting great stress on the relationship. The mother attended one of my 'Craft and Story Circles' held in the local park. She shared her 'challenge' with the group. In the next few days she wrote a story that was inspired by the miniature weaving she had started in the craft group. It was about a star that fell from the sky, and was found by a young boy in the garden. The boy wanted to help return the star to its home in the sky. He gathered coloured items from nature to weave a rainbow carpet, then he used this 'magic' carpet to fly the star back up to the sky. Afterwards the magic carpet lived with the boy under his pillow and took the boy to dream land every night to have new adventures.

Her son found a magic carpet under his pillow (in his own bed of course) the morning after his mother had told him the story. She had secretly woven it for him. Soon after this I visited the home, and the parents reported with great relief that their five-year-old now slept in his own room with the 'magic carpet' carefully placed on the table by his bed.

The tale of 'Cranky Crab' (see page 159) is another example of a story that lends itself to a prop. What better way to stop a child pinching than to wrap up the pinching fingers in warm gloves or mittens! Props can also be useful when telling stories to children. Examples of this are found in the book's storytelling section.

Focusing on specifics

A common difficulty with story making is having a theme or behaviour that is too general. My advice to beginning writers is to focus on a specific example of the behaviour you want to address. This should help to generate ideas for your story journey.

For example, for a story to help with 'aggressive' behaviour, I suggest you list specific instances of such behaviour. Perhaps you have a child who tries to push children off their chairs at meal times – the story could be about 'Mrs Chair' whose purpose in life is to be 'sat on'. The story journey could show how the chair deals with a kitten that is always pushing its brother kittens onto the floor. Perhaps the chair turns on its side or upside down until it is used properly. The chair could even have a chair rhyme or song about what a chair is meant to do. There is potential for some lovely humour here.

'Silliness', again, is too general: try to work with specific behaviour – for example trampling on flowers. Perhaps the flowers come alive and talk to the big dog that is always trampling on them. Perhaps the gardener makes a scarecrow that is befriended by the children and together they protect the garden …or the children could make a scarecrow. Children making a real scarecrow for the garden could strengthen the story.

Concentrating on specific examples should help inspire motifs for your story writing. Keep this tip in mind if you are floundering or going off at a tangent.

Adjusting stories to different situations

As a story maker, I think of myself as one of the weavers of the 'world-wide-story-web', keeping the special stories that I find, and write, alive through sharing them with others. Sometimes the sharing might need slight changes to fit a particular situation. This adds wealth to the sharing and builds the folklore of our times.

If you find a story in this book that fits your situation but needs changing somehow, do feel free to use poetic license. Remember, though, that a story is a whole entity and has its own integrity. Sometimes changing one part means you must revise and recreate the unity again.

Some of my stories have been adapted from classic tales – this is obvious in my story about 'The Three Weaver Brothers' (see page 149). Here I drew on 'The Three Little Pigs' but changed the wolf to the Kisuli-suli wind. This whirly-whirly wind can be just as devastating to the life of a bird in East Africa as the wolf was to the pigs in the classic tale.

A subtler adjustment happens every time I tell the well-loved story of 'The Star Apple' (see page 104). I always adapt the line about Grandma's cooking, depending on the community and country I am in. In the American version I say 'Sticky toffee popcorn balls', in Australia maybe 'Chocolate Lamingtons'; or in a health-conscious setting, I might say 'Carob wheat-germ balls'. In Kenya, I would say 'Mandazis', as this is a well-loved treat known to all who live in East Africa.

If you have a problem with a child who is being destructive with scissors, you could, as an example, use the existing story of 'The Pocket Knife and the Castle' (see page 119). By making a few changes you might end up with a story about 'The Scissors and the Castle', in which the boy or girl in the story dreams about shaping a beautiful castle from a large piece of card. Or it could be 'The Scissors and the Beautiful Shirt'. This could be used to motivate a sewing lesson with older children, and help create respect for craft-room equipment.

The story of 'Impatient Zebra' (see page 146), a little brown zebra who is not happy because his stripes haven't yet changed to black, has proved to be very good for helping adults realise that child development takes time – 'Good things come to those who wait!' It is a story that could easily have other animals as the central character, for example a baby swan or a young male lion that, to begin with, look quite different from the adult. This of course was also the motif underlying Hans Andersen's story 'The Ugly Duckling'.

Repetition, rhythm and rhyme

Whether you are writing a story or using one from a storybook, the therapeutic importance of repeating the story several or many times for young children (and the use of repetition and rhyme within the stories in exactly the same way each time) should not be under-estimated. It is a warm, enjoyable feeling for children to know what comes next. The rhythmic quality of repetition and rhyme provides enjoyment through familiarity and anticipation. Our children know this intuitively, and they ask for the same story, told in the same way, over and over again. This is not so different from adults who often love to hear their favourite piece of music or poetry repeated without a note or word changed.

The value of consistency and repetition as opposed to constant 'stimulation and change' is increasingly understood today as vital for young children's healthy development. Rhythm and repetition, in everyday life as well as in storytelling, help children by:

- affirming universal rhythms and continuity of life
- giving confidence and security through knowing what comes next
- developing memory and concentration skills
- developing a sense of musicality (especially when there is rhyme with the repetition)
- building language skills

As well as the benefits of repeating stories over and over again, the repetition and rhyme found within stories provide important food for children's growing souls. I encourage you in your story making to build these ingredients into your stories. This is discussed in more detail in Chapter Six. You will find many examples in the story sections of how the repetition of events and little rhymes can help create the story tension and give a musicality and flow to the story.

Happy and hope-filled endings

Both 'nursery' and 'kindergarten', mean 'garden for children'. Children can be compared to young plants in a nursery – the best way to help them grow strong is to offer as much protection as possible from the storms and winds of life.

Young children have a right to this protection – we feel this instinctively when we prevent children from watching the daily news with all its horrors of war and disasters. The wisdom of Nobel Prize Poet, Rabindranath Tagore, advises us to let children 'play on the seashore' as long as possible, untroubled by harsh realities:

On the seashore of endless worlds children meet. The infinite sky is motionless overhead and the restless water is boisterous. On the seashore of endless worlds the children meet with shouts and dances.

They build their houses with sand, and they play with empty shells. With withered leaves they weave their boats and smilingly float them on the vast deep. Children have their play on the seashore of worlds.

They know not how to swim, they know not how to cast nets. Pearl-fishers dive for pearls, merchants sail in their ships, while children gather pebbles and scatter them again.

Tempest roams in the pathless sky, ships are wrecked in the trackless water, death is abroad and children play. On the seashore of distant worlds is the great meeting of children.

This urge to protect can help us in choosing nourishing stories for young children. No matter how simple or complex the story journey, it is essential that the endings be happy and hope-filled. Good triumphing over evil is a very profound theme in folk and fairy tales, and children the world over need to hear this message.

As children reach school age (six or seven), 'consequential' stories with a just or fair ending can be introduced (see 'The Magic Fish', 'The Fisherman', and 'A Bag of Nails'). In these stories, although there is not a 'happy' ending, the main characters are not killed or hurt in any way but learn a lesson from the consequences of their negative behaviour – e.g. greed, laziness, anger. Such stories help to prepare children for real-life consequences.

Only later should we introduce the genre of stories with both unhappy and often unjust or unfair endings. Older children, in late primary school or high school, who are studying the lives of famous people, are ready to cope with the harsh reality of how Joan of Arc's life ended in being burned at the stake, or how early explorers suffered gruelling deaths through shipwrecks and starvation. Older children can cope with a sad or tragic ending. But in making your choices don't forget that teenagers, and adults too, also need the satisfaction and nourishment of a 'happy ending' from time to time. More often than not!

[i] Briefly, metaphor means seeing one thing as another, whereas simile involves a more conscious comparison of one thing with another, expressed in the word 'like'. A metaphor for a slender tree might be: 'The tree *is* a bending dancer'. The related simile, which involves somewhat more distance and detachment, would be: 'The tree is *like* a bending dancer'.

6

Different Stories for Different Ages

An enthusiastic parent rushed home after a workshop on story making and created her first therapeutic story. It was a story for bed-wetting. It had wonderful metaphors and a very creative story journey. She returned one month later to a follow-up workshop, very disappointed that her story hadn't had any effect on her child. When asked the age of her little boy, she replied, 'Almost two'!

For many years teachers and parents have been asking me to make a list of appropriate stories for different age groups, occasions and situations. This is an impossible request and one I have resisted for a good reason – stories can't be put in fixed categories. However, the above experience alerted me to the need for some kind of age-appropriate guide for story making and storytelling. This guide aims only to help you make your own decisions. Over the years, with the experience of actually writing for and telling to different age groups, one develops a 'sense' for such choices, but in the beginning the guidelines provided in this chapter may be helpful. To allow for overlapping of choices and ages, they are discussed in story genres and not in age groups.

Story rhymes and rhyming stories

Lullabies and nursery rhymes

The first 'stories' we naturally share with children are lullabies to sing a baby to sleep. Rhyming lullabies can tell a simple story –

'Sleep my little child sleep, thy father guards the sheep, thy mother shakes the dreamland tree, down falls a little dream for thee, sleep my little child sleep'.

Gentle story songs like this are not just for babies, but can be used right up to school age and older, especially if children are unwell or having nightmares. There are many traditional versions of lullabies, and it is enriching to learn new ones from other cultures. Parents / carers can also make their own lullabies – the easiest way to do this is to use a familiar tune and make up new words, especially if you are not comfortable with the original wording. For example, you might not like the breaking bough in 'Rock-a-bye baby' so you could write your own end to the song –

Rock a bye baby, in the treetops, sun filters down through green leaves above, when the wind blows the cradle will rock, and baby will sleep to cooing of doves.

Even if you don't believe you sing well, singing and chanting rhymes to your children is one of the best gifts a parent or carer can offer. With the young child so new to the world, and extremely sensitive to everything around, the real voice of the parent or carer is greatly preferable to a tape recorder. Simple body rhymes and story games come naturally into play – 'Peekaboo, I see you', 'This Little Piggy went to market', 'Round and Round the Garden'. Touch and movement, soothing words, musicality, fun and laughter, all contribute to a healthy bonding between young children and their carers.

As babies develop into toddlers, the wealth of traditional nursery rhymes (e.g. 'Twinkle, Twinkle Little Star') and nursery rhyme-type stories (e.g. 'Henny Penny'), with their wonderful rhythms, rhymes and repetition, give security and enjoyment. Children up to six years or even older can still enjoy and be nourished by their musicality and simplicity.

Story games, finger plays and body rhymes

From two–and-a-half to three onwards, with their growing awareness of their bodies and the everyday world around them, children are ready for more complex story-games (e.g. 'Here we go round the Mulberry Bush', 'Row your boat') and more detailed rhymes that tell 'body' stories (e.g. 'Heads, shoulders, knees and toes'). Finger plays are also a well-loved activity. Many little stories can be told using fingers as simple props – about a little mouse, hiding in his little house; about 'eency-weency spider' climbing the water spout; about little 'thumbkin' hiding and then coming out to say hello.

One of the main group activities in pre-schools and kindergartens is 'Ring Time' or 'Morning Ring'. This usually includes lots of different little story rhymes and story games, starting off very simply with toddlers (e.g. 'Ring-a-ring-a-roses') and progressing to the more involved actions of circle games with five- and six-year-olds (e.g. 'Round and Round the Village') and dramatising story themes through song and rhyme – e.g. harvesting food in the autumn; gathering firewood in winter; spring cleaning; summer at the beach.

Cumulative tales and nonsense stories

The three- to four-year-olds are able to absorb more complex rhyme and repetition in the form of cumulative tales. Characters in a cumulative tale keep arriving on the scene to join in with the same activity, e.g. 'The Gingerbread Man' and 'The Enormous Turnip'. These stories have plenty of repetition because each time a new character joins the tale the same action is repeated – e.g. chasing the gingerbread man, helping to pull up the turnip. Rhyming lines from the story can become everyday chants for the child. For example, to get a pre-school class to move more quickly from outside time to hand-washing time, try using 'Run, run, run as fast as you can, you can't catch me I'm the gingerbread man!'

There is also an important place for humorous and 'nonsense' stories for this pre-school age group, rich in rhyme and language – e.g. 'The Little Straw Broom' (see page 220) and 'Nibbler the Mouse'. 'Nibbler the Mouse' is a classic Russian nonsense tale about a little mouse who finds an upside-down pot and moves inside it to make it his house. Then along comes 'Croaker-the-Frog' –

Little House, Little House, who lives in this little house? I do, said Nibbler-the-Mouse, who are you? I'm Croaker-the-Frog, may I come and live with you?

Then, in progressive order, with lots of repetition, along comes 'Hare-the-Hill-Jumper', 'Reynard-the-Fox-the-Fine-Talker', 'Prowler-the-Wolf-who-Lurks-Behind-Bushes'. Then finally, 'Bear-Squash-the-Lot' comes along, sits on the pot and squashes everyone. There are many variations on this theme, including 'The Mouse and the Glove'. The animals could be substituted with others from your own environment. Nonsense stories are a genre for children that adults must be careful not to take too seriously. They speak to a child's budding sense of humour, and even defy the golden 'happy ending' rule for stories for young children – the very nature of nonsense implies 'no rules'.

Nature tales and 'everyday' stories

As concentration develops, from age three on, children can enjoy simple nature tales and 'everyday' stories – e.g. about a mother giraffe taking her baby for its first walk to the river; a tortoise that hides inside its shell whenever it meets any new animal on the path; a snail making a silver trail as it travels up and over a fence; a farmer baking a pumpkin pie; a boy going for a boat ride. Such little stories narrate simple, real and sequential events, and can often have integral rhyme and repetition. The snail may have a song she sings while slowly moving along; the farmer may chant as he bakes –

'Pumpkin pie, riddle-dum-die, delicious nutritious pumpkin pie.'
Nature tales can grow in length and complexity as the child grows
in age. An excellent tool for teachers to use in primary school when
introducing new topics of study – whether butterflies or mountains
or 'the water cycle' – a nature story can bring life to the lesson by
capturing the children's imagination from the first moment.

Another kind of 'everyday' story well-loved by pre-schoolers (and
older) is an 'I Remember When' story. If you have never told a story
to children, this is a great starting point. When working at my pre-
school in Australia, I used to recount at the lunch table a favourite
incident from a camping trip in Africa:

*I remember when I was camping in Africa. While I was eating breakfast
in front of my tent, a monkey appeared out of nowhere and took the banana off my plate. Before I could reach out to take it back the monkey had
jumped into the tree above. I looked up and saw it sitting in the fork of a
branch pealing the banana and grinning down at me.*

I recently met a little girl at the local shopping centre who had
attended my class several years before. She told me that when she
grew up she was going to Africa so a monkey could eat one of her
bananas just like in my story. I had not realised that this simple
recounting of an experience was a 'story' until this child named it
as one.

Personal 'I Remember When' stories from adults are a continual
resource for growing children, right through their childhood and
teen years and beyond. Of course these need some common-sense
censoring for young children. Starting off with innocent and simple
stories (e.g. I remember when I learnt to ride my first bicycle …) they
may slowly progress to possibly X-rated stories from one's own youth
to share with teenage and adult children at the appropriate time. I am
still 'feeding' off stories from my own grandparents – even though
they are no longer alive. I was fortunate enough to inherit some of
their diaries, and their stories of survival and resourcefulness are a rich
part of my family 'treasure chest'.

Folktales and fairytales, and the development of fantasy

As the young child grows physically and emotionally, her ability to imagine and fantasise develops. The stages of developing fantasy are best observed through changes in creative play. Whereas a younger child under two will imitate the working adult and fill a cart with blocks as mother/father fills the washing basket with clothes, the three- to four-year-old will play with and be stimulated by objects (e.g. blocks) and use them in different imaginative ways – the same block may be an iron, a car or a phone in turn, all during the same play session.

By four-and-a-half to five years, the child will usually have an imaginative idea first and then find the objects to play it out – e.g. restaurant play, hospital play, house-play, construction play (building farms, castles, boats, etc). By this stage the child's imaginative forces are blossoming and ready to be nourished by traditional folk- and fairytales.

Fairytales in the broad sense of the term, i.e. folk stories from cultures throughout the world, speak a common language that is understood by and of value to children worldwide. By dealing with universal, archetypal behaviours and situations, folktales speak to the child's budding individuality and encourage its development.

Folktales often have a 'timeless' quality. They satisfy the child's profound craving for the miraculous and offer consolation and hope. Their depth of wisdom is a healing counterweight to our materialistic age and their 'magic' makes them valuable for all children. Unlike myths that tell of the unique and miraculous deeds of gods and supernatural beings (appropriate for eight years and over), folktales and fairytales tell of people – whether lowly or highborn, a simpleton, a princess or prince, or a child. With the 'good' often pictured as 'beautiful', and 'evil' as 'ugly', the stories are about archetypes, spiritual realities, which give forms of truth other than so-called 'realistic' ones. Thoughts are transformed immediately into action; spells and transformations are soul processes so a character can suddenly become 'good', 'bewitched' or 'released'. Fairytales are like a mirror for children to see what they can become – with the witch, for example, as an image embodying all that can hamper development, and the princess or prince image embodying progressive development and the overcoming of obstacles.

In almost every tale there is either a problem that must be solved, such as the Three Billy Goats crossing the bridge, or a confrontation with evil that can take many forms, such as the wolf or hyena in 'The Three Little Pigs' or the queen in 'Snow White'. 'Tension' and 'relaxation' are integral parts of the story journey, with the different moods and challenges offering the listener a training of the soul that healthy child development needs. Often modern storybooks lack this, concentrating instead on teaching counting and the alphabet; or giving rational explanations for everyday situations (e.g. 'new baby in the house', 'first day at school'); or modifying a traditional fairytale to 'sweeten' or neutralise the ending. Children fed only on such stories may miss the opportunity for the full soul engagement developed in the overcoming of hindrances. However it is important to be aware of the right kinds of fairytales for different ages, and for this we need to investigate the following categories.

Categories of complexity

Folktales can be divided into 'categories of complexity'. In general, the gentler the theme or journey, the more appropriate the tale is for younger children, and the greater or more complex the difficulties or journey, the more appropriate it is for older children.

In seeking folktales for three- to four-year-olds, I recommend a fourfold test for their 'quality of fitness':

- Is the story full of action, in close natural sequence (more verbs than adjectives, more action than description)?
- Are the images familiar to your children (not essential, but often preferred)?
- Is the story not too long?
- Does the story include rhyme and repetition (not essential, but preferred)?

Examples of such stories include 'The Enormous Turnip' (Russian); 'Goldilocks and the Three Bears' (English); 'The Three Billy Goats Gruff' (Norwegian – see page 181).

The next category, suitable for the four-and-a-half to six-year-olds, includes many of the tales that we normally associate with the term 'fairytale'. These stories can still be tested as above, but contain more challenges and more detail, with an overall cheerful mood without too much sorrow or struggle. Although obstacles are encountered they do not weigh too heavily on the soul of the listener.

Examples include 'The Elves and the Shoemaker' (see page 226); 'Rhodopese' (Egyptian – see page 185); 'Tiddalick' (Indigenous Australian); 'The Antelope, the Butterfly and the Chameleon' (Kikuyu – see page 224); 'The Fisherman' (East African – see page 151).

Six- to seven-year-olds enjoy and benefit from stories of increasing length, challenge and detail, with characters that have a personal experience of suffering or sorrow. The confrontation with evil may be stronger and more challenging, and there may be more twists and turns along the journey.

Examples include: 'Snow White' and 'The Seven Ravens' (Grimm); 'Garden of Light' (see page 127); 'Akimba and the Magic Cow' (African – see page 114); 'The Invisible Hunter' (American Indian – see page 181).

For the eight-year-olds and over, besides more complex folktales from many cultures, a recommended story-centred curriculum for home and school is the one followed in the Steiner education model. In progressive classes this covers the Norse myths, African, Persian, Indian and Egyptian stories, and the Greek and Roman legends. Teachers also write their own pedagogical stories to introduce educational content and concepts such as teaching the alphabet. Such stories can help turn 'stones' into 'bread', dry facts into life-filled pictures, transforming what might otherwise be tedious into an inspirational experience. Stories and storytelling methods are also used to address challenging behaviour and children's social and emotional development. In Steiner schools, teachers and children experience the wisdom and power of such stories as an integral, daily part of education.[i]

Such a story-centred curriculum can develop children's imagination, helping them grow into 'juicy plums' as adults and preventing the 'dried-up prune' syndrome mentioned in Chapter 1. I encourage all parents, therapists and teachers to find ways to bring this wealth of stories from our mythological history into children's lives, along with those we creatively devise ourselves. Through the light of stories we can nourish and help our children develop into imaginative, well-rounded young adults, ready to carry our world into a positive future.

i   See, for example: L. Francis Edmunds, *Introduction to Steiner Education: The Waldorf School* (details in reference section)

7

Truth and Morality

Is it true?

Whether telling stories of your own, or stories from folk culture, it is important to consider the question of 'truth' and stories. Some people are concerned that folk fairy tales do not render truthful pictures of life and are therefore unhealthy. Psychologist Bettelheim states that the truth of fairy stories is that of the imaginative realm, rather than ordinary causality. Fairy tales are about archetypes, spiritual realities, which give forms of truth other than so-called 'realistic' ones.

I was once privileged to listen to an American storyteller called 'Floating Eagle Feather'. He began his story session with an open question:

Some people believe the world is made of atoms. I believe the world is made of stories. What do you believe?

Before writing or telling a children's story, the storyteller needs to know what she believes. As you tell a story a child will subtly sense whether you yourself are really 'inside' and 'behind' it, or are only 'making something up' that you are not fully connected with.

For an answer to the child's question, 'Is it true?' many fairytales offer an answer to this in the first line of the story. Beginnings such as 'Once upon a time ...' and 'In olden times, when wishing still helped.....' make it clear that the stories take place on a different level from everyday reality. If children persist with asking whether a story is true, Nancy Mellon, an experienced storyteller, suggests one could simply say, 'Let's listen to the story again'. Or the answer might sometimes be, in a mood of wonder, 'I think this story is truer than true!'

Nature research

When writing a nature tale, getting the facts right is important. If the wind in your story is blowing across a rainbow bridge, and the colours of the rainbow need to be mentioned, then be careful to describe the correct colour order (unless, of course, the story is about a mixed-up rainbow!). If writing a story about a baby wombat, it helps to do some research into how it enters its mother's pouch from under and behind, not in front like all the other marsupials. An Australian colleague of mine made this mistake in a wombat story and a child in the class corrected her. Since this time she has been careful to research her nature tales more thoroughly.

Ideas for writing stories can be greatly enriched through observation and research. Important and fascinating facts on the habitat, diet and characteristics of animals and birds can help generate new ideas for the story journey. All my fauna- and flora-based stories have been created from research combined with, where possible, my own observations of the particular animal, tree or flower. Observing that the stalk of a pumpkin is attached to the vegetable in a star-like shape gave me the idea for including a dream about a star in my 'Pumpkin Munchkin' story (see page 173). My research on whale songs motivated my choice of a whale for a story on whingeing (whining) behaviour (see page 100).

Fibs, lies and tall tales

Most dictionaries define a storyteller, firstly, as someone who tells or writes stories, and secondly, as someone who tells fibs or lies. There is definitely an interesting connection between telling stories and telling lies. Lying or bragging contests can bring out wonderful storytellers, and for some of us who have never told a story before, telling a 'tall tale' can often be the easiest way to have our first go. The word 'fiction' of course, means something that is not strictly true – and without it our culture would be immeasurably poorer. The life of the imagination conjures a multitude of scenarios which, while not materially true, may nevertheless express spiritual truth. They are indeed often 'truer than true'.

Most, if not all human beings tell lies in one way or another. Some brand their lies 'white lies' to justify their use. Others never let the truth get in the way of a good story, and embellish a travelling tale to keep their listeners attentive for longer. Fishermen have the reputation for bragging about 'the one that got away'.

I think everyone would agree, however, that for healthy emotional and social development children need to learn about the consequences of lying, both 'white lies' and serious lying. Children also need to learn how to let their conscience be their guide, something that is not by any means an overnight process. Awareness of a moral aspect to one's conduct, together with a preference for right over wrong, is one of the most important outcomes of a truly holistic education. The 'fictions' of storytelling are actually a wonderful aid in this process throughout childhood.

Truth is such a vital subject for our time, especially given the corruption in so many leading institutions and government bodies. Children can learn to lie at such an early age: perhaps as a protective tendency, or as a game and experience from which they get quite a thrill. It is sometimes difficult for parents and teachers to know how to sort out lies while still honouring children's imagination.

One helpful hint that I learnt from my teaching years is to be careful not to jump in and label 'lies' as 'lies' when children are very young. For pre-school children the adult's role should be to show by example, and to find ways to gently lead a 'lie' back to truth, not to quickly 'set it in concrete' by labelling it. For example, when a child tells the group about his travel adventures at the weekend (and the teacher knows the child was really at home both days) she could say 'Thank you for your story, Dylan', and not 'That is a lie Dylan, you know you were home all weekend'. This way the teacher is simply acknowledging that the child had a need to make up a story, perhaps to match other children's exciting weekend stories. Of course, if Dylan's habit of making up 'bragging' stories persists, the teacher may need to discuss it with the parent and find out the deeper reasons behind this – it may be a behaviour he has developed at home to get the attention of his busy parents or impress his older siblings.

Another situation that often arises with pre-schoolers is when a child says to the teacher, 'I don't have anything in my pocket' when really the teacher knows he has just pocketed a favourite little toy from the classroom. Instead of the teacher labelling this a lie, a gentler yet still effective approach is to simply put a hand into the child's pocket and say, 'Goodness me, a little toy has jumped in here. Can you help me put it back in its home?' In this way the teacher is leading the child into 'right action' and the child should feel much better for this, hopefully learn from it; and will certainly appreciate not being labelled!

Great care still needs to be taken once children are school age. It is best not to discuss the lie or theft in front of the whole group, but to take the child aside for a quiet chat. Nancy Mellon uses the metaphor of a 'thorn' when giving advice on dealing with a lying or stealing child. She believes that dishonest deeds are carried like a thorn inside the child, and direct exposure can push the thorn deeper rather than releasing it.

This leads to the use of stories. Stories have the potential to help the thorn find its way out. By leaving the listener free to come to his own conclusion, stories can feed the growing conscience in a nourishing and wholesome way.

Every culture has developed stories to teach the consequences of dishonesty. The Grimm's story, 'The Wolf and the Seven Kids' shows that lying does not get you what you want. A South African Xhosa tale with the same theme is transcribed in this book (see page 108). In both stories, the wolf or hyena, pretending to be the mother, repeatedly lies to the children in order to get inside their house.

The lovable Italian story of the wooden doll Pinocchio, whose nose grew longer with every lie he told, has a powerful message here for children who have a serious lying habit, as does the classic story of 'The Boy Who Cried Wolf'.

Lying contests and the use of humour

To address the theme of lying with older children in a light-hearted way, a teacher or family member could introduce the idea of holding a lying contest, or a contest of 'tall tales'. Dividing into small groups, one child can act as the judge and the other two can compete with a false story or tall tale. The theme could be as simple as 'What I did last weekend' or 'What happened to me on the way home from school yesterday'. If there are enough contestants, you could start with heats and lead up to semi-finals and a final.

Lying contests can generate a lot of fun. They also help create awareness of the difference between truth and falsehoods, and the appropriate time and place for both.

Telling lies for entertainment has been an accepted part of many cultures for hundreds of years. In parts of Africa, and America's deep South, lying contests are part of the folk history of black people. There are also records from Anglo-Saxon times of a tradition called 'Lying for the Whetstone'. Apparently an old Whitsun custom, it has been celebrated in England since the 14th century. He who could tell the greatest lie was rewarded with a whetstone to 'sharpen his wit'.

'Tall Tales' have their origin in the bragging contests that often occurred when the rough folk of frontier communities gathered. A uniquely American or Australian story form, they usually feature a larger-than-life, or superhuman, main character with a specific task, and a problem that is solved in a humorous or outrageous way. Tall tales and lying contests have appealing use for primary children – both telling existing tales and writing new ones.

Moral or moralistic?

For thousands of years, as we have seen, cultures worldwide have been using the medium of story to teach morals and values. Many traditional folk stories have moral qualities, and the listener receives these in different ways. This is all part of the nature and 'power' of story. In writing or choosing stories, it is important to be aware of the difference between a moral tale and a 'moralistic' or cautionary one. A moral tale, through an imaginative story journey, should leave the listener free to come to his own conclusion.

The delightful African tale, 'Akimba and the Magic Cow' (see page 114), is an example of a story journey with moral qualities. Dishonesty has its consequences and the thief ends up with a 'beating stick' fourth time round instead of a cow that produced gold coins, a sheep that produced silver coins, or a chicken that laid eggs. Because of the story structure, with its repetition of events, by the time the stick is introduced the listener is hoping for a change, ready for a change, wanting a change! And how delightful that the final sequence is humorous, that a serious message about dishonesty can be delivered through the medium of humour.

The listener has a similar experience in the folktale of 'The Magic Fish' (see page 136). The wife is greedy and keeps wishing to own more and more – a house, a mansion, a castle, the sun and the moon! To the great relief of the listener she ends up losing everything and is back in her little shack on the beach at the end of the story. In the words of one of my sons, sighing with relief at the end of the story, 'She wanted too much!'

A moralistic tale, however, is more like a sermon or lecture disguised as a story. Such a story was once written by a teacher to encourage good manners in her class. This story was about a child whom no one wanted to play with because he didn't say please or thank you. Then he learnt to say please and thank you and the children wanted to play with him. Her words seemed more like a lecture or a direct instruction. They lacked the metaphoric and journey qualities of a story.

For a story to help children come to their own moral conclusions, usually some kind of imaginative journey is required. There seems to be a definite need for 'indirectness'. A story is in danger of being moralistic when the purpose is too obvious. I can usually tell the moralistic ones by the way they make me feel a little squeamish at the end. In contrast a good moral tale leaves me feeling well satisfied, like a nourishing meal. But how I receive and react to a story may be very different from you. I only put these thoughts on paper to get you thinking, if you are planning to write your own therapeutic stories.

Most importantly, whatever stories you choose to write and tell, be careful not to end them by giving the children a summary of *your* perception of the moral values. Leave the listeners free to come to their own conclusions – trust in the power of the story!

8

Story Making Exercises

The following exercises are taken from workshop discussions. Each one includes the outline of a story journey for you to try to add metaphoric 'clothes' and finish the story. These are suggestions only. The stories could be written with many different choices of metaphor and journey.

The Kangaroo Brothers

A story idea to reduce fighting and aggressive behaviour in a group of six- and seven-year-olds. The kangaroo has been chosen as an obvious metaphor – kangaroos love to box and fight!

- Two kangaroos live alone on the grassy plains
- One day they meet and at first they are friends
- Then they start to fight – kick and box! (suggested use of lots of repetition here, with several examples of the fighting – when, where and how)
- One day a fire starts in the bush and sweeps across the grassy plains (or the river floods the land?).
- The two kangaroos use their boxing hands for positive work – together they carry the little animals out of the burnt grasslands and across the river to safety (or out of the flood and up into the high country?)
- Alternatively, instead of using a fire or flood in the story, you could bring in the idea of many thorns starting to grow in the grasslands and the kangaroos become like 'bush doctors', using their hands to pull thorns out of animal paws, birds' feet, lizards' feet, etc. You need to make the final decision on what obstacle and helping metaphors to use here.

- After this the kangaroos occasionally enjoy a box or a fight, but most of the time they are too busy doing other things (give examples of activities related to your chosen story journey)

The Two Pigeons

A story idea for building self-confidence in a shy five-year-old girl.

- Two pigeons, one brave and adventurous and one shy and cowardly
- The shy bird is always relying on his friend to be the leader and tell him what to do (build up the story by working in some obstacle metaphors here – giving examples of when, where and how)
- One day the shy pigeon is watching from his perch and sees a cat sneaking up on some baby birds in a nearby tree
- The shy pigeon looks for his friend to help with advice, but his friend is not around
- The shy pigeon finds a way to scare off the cat (use a helping metaphor here) and save the baby birds – this idea needs to be expanded and given detail.
- The baby birds are safe, their mother returns to thank the 'hero' pigeon who is now feeling more confident

Mrs. Table and the Chair Children

This idea of a humorous story arose when I visited a playgroup where the teacher was struggling to get the three and four-year-old children to come to the table for morning tea (morning break or 'elevenses' in the UK). Until this new teacher arrived, the children had been allowed to eat their snacks anywhere and anytime and had had no experience of a group mealtime. Something creative was needed to help ease in a new routine.

- Mrs Table and the Chair Children live in a schoolroom but are always lonely – nobody ever uses them!
- One day they decide to try different ways to attract the children to them (helping metaphors needed here). Perhaps the Chair Children waddle out to the garden and pick some flowers to

bring back to make Mrs Table more attractive, and/or the Chair Children start to rock backwards and forwards in a dance to make the children notice them.

- Think of one or two more things that could happen at this point to make the table and/or chairs appealing. Or perhaps the story is already long enough for the age group?
- Finally Mrs Table and the Chair Children could sing a song. The children hear their music, delight in the song, and one by one come to the table (repeat song several times, and use at morning tea everyday).

Morning tea, morning tea,
Time to come and sit with me,
With drink to drink and food to eat,
Time to come and rest your feet!

SECTION THREE

STORIES FOR CHALLENGING BEHAVIOUR

This section spans a collection of fifty-two stories for commonly identified forms of behaviour. To help you find your way, the pages are organised into the following categories with suggested stories for various, numerous possibilities. These categories have been arbitrarily chosen for easy referencing – I definitely don't recommend using them as 'labels' for behaviour.

- Bored / whingeing
- Dishonest / sneaky
- Disrespectful / uncaring
- Greedy / unable to share
- Irritating / impatient
- Lazy
- Pinching / hurting / fighting
- Shy / introverted
- Noisy / disruptive
- Teasing / bullying
- Uncooperative
- Wild / restless

The stories are from my own writing collection as well as wisdom tales from other cultures, in particular African cultures. Some stories have already been used (with different degrees of success) and have notes documenting their use. Others have been newly written or transcribed for this book. Any correspondence from the use of these stories and/or any of your own therapeutic stories are welcome (see my website at back of book).

The stories are mainly suitable for children aged three to eight, although some have been used successfully with teenagers and adults. Before each story are notes indicating suggested ages and use. In general, the shorter, simpler and more repetitive the story, the more suitable it is for younger ones. The longer and more complex the plot, the more it is suitable for late kindergarten and primary ages ('Different stories for different ages' is explored in more detail in Chapter Six).

The suggested stories are the tip of the iceberg of possibilities. With the help of the section on 'Therapeutic Story Writing', I hope you will explore many more ideas.

9

Bored or Whingeing

Bored Baboon

This story was written for children five years old and over. With the message of the importance and fun of 'play', it has also been used in parent education courses as a springboard for discussion. I have experienced that in dealing with behaviour challenges (e.g. boredom) we so often need to reach the adults as well as the children.

Mtoto Baboon was bored. She didn't want to play with her friends. That's BORING, she would say. She didn't want to climb trees. That's BORING, she would say. She didn't want to go and splash in the river. That's BORING, she would say. Mtoto Baboon seemed to just want to hang around being bored and she was driving her mother crazy with her boredom.

So Mother Baboon decided to call in old wise Grandfather Baboon to talk to Mtoto and sort out the BORING problem. Grandfather Baboon sat down with Mtoto and made some suggestions. But Mtoto was bored with her grandfather's ideas. She didn't want to throw pebbles off the cliffs. That's BORING, she said. She didn't want to swing on the long vines. That's BORING, she said. She didn't want to roll through the tall grass. That's BORING, she said.

Then Grandfather Baboon asked her what she really wanted to do. This was a very difficult question for Mtoto, for you see, she didn't really know the answer. But of course, she didn't want to admit this, so she said, 'I just want to sit by myself and do nothing'. And then she ran off from her grandfather, and followed a path into the thick bushes, looking for a comfortable place to sit by herself and do nothing.

As she was running through the bushes, she noticed a box-kind-of-thing next to a tall tree on the edge of the path. It had a smooth floor and a flat roof, and shiny bars all around the sides. And in the front there was a little door, just large enough for her to fit through. And best of all, on the floor at the back, there was a ripe golden banana. Mtoto Baboon's favourite food!

'This looks like a comfortable house to sit in by myself and do nothing', thought Mtoto to herself. And without hesitating she stepped inside, sat down on the floor and started to eat the banana. As she picked it up to take her first bite, the door of the little house slammed shut. At first this didn't worry Mtoto Baboon, as she was so happy enjoying her golden banana.

By the time she had finished eating Mtoto was feeling tired. So she curled up on the smooth floor and fell fast asleep. She slept for a long time, and when she woke up she was quite stiff and sore. She tried to stretch her long baboon arms and legs, but there was not enough room in this little house for moving and stretching. Next she tried to push open the door so she could go outside to stretch. It was then that she realised that the little house was not a house, but a trap, and the door was locked tight.

All baboons were told at an early age about hunters and their traps, but in her hurry to run away from her grandfather, Mtoto had completely forgotten this vitally important warning.

Oh how Mtoto Baboon wished she had listened to her elders! Suddenly their ideas of climbing trees and playing by the river and swinging on vines seemed like the best things in the world that a child baboon could hope to do! But now, Mtoto could not go anywhere or do anything. Trembling inside the trap, she waited for the dreaded sound of the hunter to return.

Mtoto did not have to wait long. Stamp, stamp, stamp, came the hunter's boots along the path. Louder and louder the stamping grew, until the boots were right outside the bars, and two long arms were bending down to pick up the trap.

Suddenly Mtoto heard a loud barking and quick as a flash, she saw a large baboon with strong white teeth come swinging down out of the tree next to the trap. The baboon gave the hunter such a fright that he dropped the trap and ran away as fast as his long hunters' legs could carry him. As the trap hit the ground, the lock fell apart and the door swung open.

Mtoto quickly jumped out and landed right in the arms of the baboon who had saved her. She looked into his face and saw it was her very own grandfather.

'Grandfather, you are not only wise, but you are strong and brave as well,' cried Mtoto. 'I want to grow up to be just like you.'

'Well', laughed her grandfather with his deep baboon laugh, 'you had better run off and join your friends in their play, as playing will make you strong and wise and brave too.'

Mtoto gave her grandfather a big baboon hug, and then ran off to join her friends in their game by the river.

And from that day to this, Mtoto Baboon was never bored again.

So if you go into the African bushland, you may be lucky enough to see Mtoto with her friends, climbing trees, splashing in the river, throwing pebbles off the cliffs, swinging on the long vines and rolling through the tall grass – having fun from morning to night.

Whingeing (Whining) Whale

Dealing with persistent (and often annoying) whingeing and whining behaviour is a universal challenge, especially for parents who have

24-hour, 7-days-per-week involvement with young children.

The story of Whingeing Whale has been used with ages four years and upwards by a cross-cultural group, from a teacher in Cape Town, to a mother in the slums of Nairobi, to a psychologist in Byron Bay (who is using the story with adults in personal growth counselling). Each time it has had encouraging results, especially with young children when the message is strengthened by the repeated use of the poem. The teacher in Cape Town found it necessary to use a musical pipe to blow some deep notes at the end of the story – her children insisted on hearing what beautiful whale-song really sounded like!

There was once a little whale who did nothing all day long but whine and whinge to his mother. No matter what mother whale did or how hard she tried to please her young one, nothing was ever quite right. She was swimming too fast or too slow, the water was too hot or too cold, his dinner was too much or not enough.

All day long, Whingeing Whale just swam around his mother in their ocean home, chanting his whingeing song:

> *I don't like this and I don't like that,*
> *I don't want this and I don't want that,*
> *I can't do this and I can't do that, my life is no good any way!*

Mother Whale tried to teach her baby the beautiful whale songs that young whales need to learn if they are going to grow up and have families of their own. But Whingeing Whale was too busy chanting his whingeing song to take any notice of learning silly old whale songs.

> *I don't like this and I don't like that,*
> *I don't want this and I don't want that,*
> *I can't do this and I can't do that, my life is no good any way!*

Mother Whale tried to get her baby to play with the other young whales in the ocean. But Whingeing Whale didn't want to be bothered. And the other young whales in the whale pod were tired of listening to Whingeing Whale and didn't particularly want to play with him either. His loud whingeing noises were spoiling their ocean home.

One day, as all the whales were swimming near the coastline, they started to move out to sea to reach deeper waters. But Whingeing

Whale had been so busy whingeing that he didn't notice that all the other whales, including his mother, had changed direction. He continued swimming straight ahead, and before he knew what was happening, he had crossed the coastal reef and found himself in a small lagoon.

Then the tide started to turn, and the water in the lagoon slowly started to empty out through the reef passage. Whingeing Whale was left stranded in the shallows, with the water only just covering his whale back, and getting lower and lower with every passing moment.

What was he to do? It was no use chanting his whingeing song as his mother wasn't around to hear him. Then, deep in his whale memory, he heard the most beautiful sounds. He listened and then tried to repeat them. At first his singing was very weak, but the more he tried, the stronger his voice grew. Soon he was booming out a song, a most beautiful whale song.

The song travelled through the water, over the reef, and out into the deep ocean. The song travelled all the way to where his mother and the other whales were swimming. As soon as the whale pod heard the young whale calling, all the whales turned around and swam back towards the reef. As they swam, they leapt high out of the water, and back down again, and up again, and down again. And as they leapt up and splashed down, they made a giant wave roll on ahead of them. When they reached the reef they stopped and waited. The giant wave rolled over the rocks and filled the lagoon with enough water to help the stranded whale swim out to safety. He found his whale pod waiting for him on the other side of the reef, and was escorted back to their deep ocean home.

His mother was so proud of her young one. 'At last you have learnt the power and beauty of our whale song' she whispered to him. And she swam around him and nuzzled him all over his body with her whale snout – which is how mother whales kiss and hug their children.

Of course, the young whale was very happy to be back safe and sound with his whale pod. And now he knew how to use his whale voice to sing such beautiful songs, he never bothered to whinge and whine again. In fact, he made up a new whale song to teach his friends. If you are ever swimming in the ocean and listen very carefully, you may also hear this beautiful song:

I can sing this and I can sing that, I enjoy this and I enjoy that,
I can do this and I can do that, my life is so good every day!

The Squeaky Bed

A universal story for all ages to help re-evaluate how good or bad things are in life. Especially valuable to use when a child is continually complaining about something trivial.

I have used this with large groups of mixed-age children and also with adults at conferences – to get them laughing and actively involved. For the adults it has helped provide 'healing' entertainment at the end of an intense day or week of thinking and concentration. The story lends itself to the storyteller dividing the audience into 'animal' sections and then, as each animal enters the house, there can be much noise and activity as this is acted out. The comparison between the small squeaky noise (made by a chosen member of the audience) and all the animals making their cacophony of sounds is remarkable!

There was once an old woman who lived on a farm. She was very content with her life except for one thing – she didn't like her squeaky bed. All through the night it made so many different squeaks and noises that she was finding it hard to sleep.

It happened that one night the squeaks grew so loud it was more than she could bear. The next day she went to visit the wise man in the village and told him her problem. The wise man sent her back to her farm and told her to bring the cow in to live in the house.

'Very strange advice' thought the old woman, 'but he is the wise man so I will do as he says'.

On reaching home, she called the cow inside, and that evening, as well as the bed squeaking, the cow was also mooing all night long.

Back went the old woman to the wise man, and this time he advised her to go back to her farm and bring in the sheep.

[The story goes on and on, until her house is filled with all her farm animals – cow, sheep, donkey, pig, rooster, etc. all making their respective noises through the night (the list can be as long or short as the concentration span of the listeners)].

Finally the old woman couldn't stand it any longer. She had a terrible headache and she hadn't slept for weeks. She returned to the wise man and told him that she was going to tell all the villagers that he really couldn't be a 'wise man' as he had given such unhelpful, silly advice.

The wise man begged the old woman to accept one last piece of advice from him – 'Go home old woman, take all the animals out of your house and let them go back to where they belong'.

The old woman went home and put the cow, sheep, donkey, pig, rooster, etc. out of her house. That night, and all the following nights, she slept deeply and soundly.

The Star Apple

This story is of unknown origins and is re-written by the author. It is suitable for all ages. It is a positive example of how a child's boredom can be turned into a wonder-filled adventure, with the first stimulus coming from a creative parent. When I tell this story I usually cut an apple (horizontally, not from stalk to base). I then put the two halves together, and hide them in a cloth in my lap, ready to open and show the star to the listeners at the appropriate time.

There was once a little boy who was tired of all his picture books, tired of all his puzzles and tired of all his toys.

'What should I do?' he asked his mother.

Now this little boy's mother always knew beautiful things for little boys to do, and she said 'You should go on a journey and look for a little red house, with no windows and no doors – and a star hiding inside'.

Well, the little boy's eyes grew wide with excitement. 'But Mother, where could I find such a house?' he said.

'Down the lane, past the farmer's house, and up the hill – but be sure when you find it, to bring it back to show me.'

So the little boy set out. It was a beautiful day – the sun was shining, the sky was blue and he was so happy to be going on an adventure. He skipped down the lane, singing to himself. He hadn't gone far when he saw the farmer standing outside his big brown barn looking out over his fields of grain and corn.

'Excuse me, farmer,' said the little boy, 'can you tell me where I could find a little red house, with no windows and no doors – and a star hiding inside?'

'Well,' said the farmer, 'I've lived here a good many years and I don't know of such a house. You should ask Grandma – Grandma knows how to knit red mittens and Grandma knows how to make sticky toffee popcorn balls. Grandma will surely know.'

The little boy continued down the lane looking for Grandma's house. Soon he came to where Grandma was sitting on her rocking chair in the middle of her garden of herbs and marigolds.

'Excuse me, Grandma,' said the little boy, 'can you tell me where I could find a little red house, with no windows and no doors – and a star hiding inside?'

'Oh,' sighed Grandma, 'I should like to know of such a house myself – it would be warm when the nights are cold, and the star would make a beautiful light. You should ask the Wind – the Wind blows over the hills and through the valleys, the Wind blows all around the world, the Wind knows all the secrets.'

So the little boy continued on his journey, looking for the Wind. He started to climb up a hill and he hadn't gone far when down the hill to meet him came the Wind. It blew once around his head, once more and once again.

'Excuse me, Wind' said the little boy, 'can you tell me where I could find a little red house, with no windows and no doors – and a star hiding inside'.

Well, the Wind laughed, and seemed to say, 'Follow me'. It blew to the top of the hill to where an apple tree stood. It blew once around the apple tree, once more and once again. It blew an apple off a branch to land in the grass below.

When the little boy reached the top of the hill he bent down and picked up the apple. He held it in his hands and looked at it carefully. It was as round and red as the sun had been able to paint it. It had no windows and no doors. It had a little stalk on top that looked just like a chimney.

'I wonder' said the little boy, and from out of his pocket he took his pocket-knife and cut the apple right across the middle.

When he opened the two halves, he saw, hiding inside … a star!

'Thank you Wind,' said the little boy.

'You're welcome,' whispered the Wind.

And the little boy carried his little red house, with no windows and no doors – and a star hiding inside – all the way home to show his mother.

The Secret of Easter

This story is a positive example of how finding an answer to a riddle can turn a 'boring' nothing-to-do-day into a wonder-filled adventure. As it is quite long, I suggest it is suitable for age five and upwards.

There once lived a little boy who longed to know the secret of Easter. Every year when the hot summer days were cooling down and a white cloud blanket was covering the sky, he knew Easter was coming soon. In his country Easter always came with the clouds and the rain. He would hear his Mother and Father talking about Easter, he would hear his big brother and sister talking about Easter, he knew Easter was coming, he could feel Easter was coming…but he didn't really understand what Easter was.

'Mummy' he would often ask, 'What is Easter?'

'Ah, my child', his Mother would say, 'Easter is a very special secret.'

'Mummy, who will tell me this secret?'

'Only Father Sun can tell you such a special secret, and he will tell you when he is ready to tell you.' And his Mother would go on with her work.

The little boy would run outside and look up to where Father Sun was smiling down through windows in the white cloud blanket, and he would listen, and wait, and listen, and wait. This year he was waiting and wishing more than ever that Father Sun would tell him the Easter Secret.

One morning he woke very early. Something felt different today – the birds seemed to be singing to him, the sunbeams dancing through his window seemed to be beckoning him outside. He rose and dressed himself and without even waiting to have breakfast he ran outside into the garden. The sky was filled with clouds, but over in the East was a great window and Father Sun was shining right through. He seemed to be reaching his sunbeam arms right out to the little boy and the little boy reached his arms up to meet the sunbeams. He listened and waited, and listened and waited, and then he heard this message from Father Sun…

The secret you seek, in a little house I keep,
Where my golden light, shines day and night.

He listened again….

The secret you seek, in a little house I keep,
Where my golden light, shines day and night.

The little boy was so happy to know at last where to find the secret. He ran here and there and everywhere around the garden, but soon realised it was not going to be so easy to find this little house, where the Sun's golden light shines both day and night.

'I know, I'll ask the Wind, he blows all over the land, surely he will know where to find this little house,' and he ran down to where the wind was blowing around the bushes at the bottom of the garden.

'Wind, Wind, dear friend Wind, can you tell me where I can find the little house, where the Sun's golden light shines day and night?'

But the Wind was too busy blowing. 'Ask Tree,' said Wind.

So the little boy ran to where the great fig tree grew in the middle of the garden.

'Tree, Tree, dear friend Tree, can you tell me where I can find the little house where the Sun's golden light shines day and night?'

But Tree was too busy growing. 'Ask Ant,' said Tree.

So the little boy ran to where the ant holes were, in the middle of the rockery.

'Ant, Ant, dear friend Ant, can you tell me where I can find the little house where the Sun's golden light shines day and night?'

But Ant was too busy scurrying. 'Ask Bee,' said Ant.

So the little boy ran to where the flowers grew by the back wall of the house.

'Bee, Bee, dear friend Bee, can you tell me where I can find the little house where the Sun's golden light shines day and night?'

But Bee was too busy buzzing.

Just when the little boy was beginning to wonder if he would ever find this little house, where the Sun's golden light shines day and night, he heard his Mother calling him for breakfast.

He ran inside, washed his hands, and sat up at the table. 'I'll ask my Mother,' he thought. So he told her about the message from Father Sun. 'I've looked and looked everywhere, and I've asked the Wind and I've asked the Tree, I've asked the Ant, and I've asked the Bee. Can you tell me where I can find the little house where the Sun's golden light shines day and night?'

His Mother smiled a very warm smile and said: 'Why, it's right in front of you.'

The little boy looked down and there, right in front of him, in a little wooden egg-cup, was a smooth, round, shiny, egg-house. His Mother helped him cut it open and inside, cradled in a soft white bed, was a ball of golden light, shining day and night.

The little boy was so happy to find the Easter Secret, and so hungry after his busy searching, that he ate up all his breakfast and one *extra* hot cross bun, and then ran out into the garden to play. And as he played he sang to himself:

> *A white cloud blanket is wrapping around,*
> *A secret hiding down on the ground,*
> *A secret hiding in a soft straw nest,*
> *An Easter secret that we love the best.*

10

Dishonest or Sneaky

The Doves and the Hyena

A traditional Xhosa story researched by Maria Msebenzi and re-written by the author. This story has a similar theme to the Grimm's fairytale, 'The Wolf and the Seven Kids'. It addresses the themes of lying and deceit and is suitable for age six and upwards.

A long time ago in the middle of a forest there lived a mother dove. She had her nest at the top of a green leafy tree, and in her nest there were three baby doves.

Every day the mother dove would leave the nest to search for food. Before she flew away, she would remind her children not to open the door of the nest and not to throw the rope out to anyone else except her. The children would know when she returned as they would hear her singing her mother-dove song.

Every day the children would wait inside their nest with the door safely closed. When their mother returned, she would stand at the bottom of the tree and sing. The children would then open the door and throw the rope out for their mother to climb up with their food.

One day the mother dove had returned to her tree and was singing up to her children. Without her knowing it, her singing was overheard by a hungry hyena. He watched as the door of the nest opened and the baby doves threw down the rope and the mother dove climbed up.

The hyena thought how much he would love to have those baby doves for his dinner. So he devised a cunning plan. He waited until mother dove had left the nest the next morning, then he stood at the bottom of the tree and tried to sing. But his song was very coarse. Even when he tried to squeeze his voice to be softer, the baby doves knew it was not their mother and would not open the door and throw down the rope.

The hyena decided to find an apple to soften his voice. He quickly went to a near-by farm and picked a green apple from the orchard. He chewed and chewed and swallowed the apple, even though it tasted quite bitter. Then he went back to the tree and tried to sing again.

But his song was still quite coarse, and even when he tried to squeeze his voice to be softer, the baby doves knew it was not their mother and would not open the door and throw down the rope.

By now the hyena was getting quite angry. He ran back to the farm and frightened the farmer into giving him one of his special red apples that grew on an apple tree right next to the farmhouse. When the hyena chewed and swallowed the red apple, the sweet juices helped to soften and sweeten his voice. He returned to the forest and once again stood at the bottom of the tree and sang to the baby doves. This time the little doves thought it really was their mother returning home. They opened the door and threw down the rope.

Quickly and quietly the hyena started to climb up the rope. He climbed and climbed until he was almost at the nest. Just then the mother dove returned to the tree. She saw what was happening and sang to her children, 'My beautiful children, quickly close the door'!

Hearing their mother's voice, the children let go of the rope and quickly climbed back inside their nest, closing the door behind them. The hyena rolled and tumbled, all the way down to the ground, landing with a loud thud and hurting his back.

Since this time the hyena has always loped along with a broken back. And the mother dove has never left her children alone in the house again. As soon as they are old enough, she teaches them to fly and find food for themselves.

Dishonest Dingo

This story has been written for seven- to nine-year-olds (a rough age-guide). It has quite strong themes and metaphors. These have been necessary to help address the seriousness of stealing.[i] The story introduces the positive effect of listening to one's conscience in the transforming journey from dishonesty to honesty. The story could be used for five- and six year-olds, but is definitely not appropriate for the under-fours. This younger age group comprehend borrowing and 'taking home to show mum', but not stealing!

On the red dusty plains in the middle of a wide land, there once lived a dingo called Little D. He had been born in a litter of many dingo pups and was the last and smallest of all his brothers. But whereas his brothers wore yellow coats there was something different about him ... he was shining white!

Because he was the smallest, and because he looked so different, he always had to fight for what he needed. As a baby pup, he had to learn to scramble over all the other pups and push his way through to drink some milk from his mother. Then, as he grew older, he would always be fighting to get any part of the hunt that his father dragged home. He would also have to fight and wrestle to get any spare bones to bury for food another day.

Most of the time, Little D, the smallest and whitest dingo, fought a losing battle with his brothers and never was able to get enough to eat. The constant fighting for food led this young dingo into dishonest ways. He discovered it was easier to steal his food rather than fight for it.

It all happened like this.

One day Little D was rolling in the red dust of the plains and one of his brothers walked by with a large bone in his mouth. To Little D's amazement the brother didn't notice him. Because Little D was so covered with dust he blended into the surrounding red plains.

Little D stopped rolling in the dust and started to follow his brother. Into the scrub his brother carried the bone, and once amongst the bushes, he dug a deep hole and buried it.

When the brother had returned to the plains, Little D dug up the bone and took it away to enjoy as his own.

The next day, Little D rolled in the red dust and waited for the next brother to come by with his bone to bury. Again, he followed him – this time to a rocky hill near the scrublands. The brother with the bone then dug a hole amongst the rocks and put the bone inside. Once the brother had returned to the plains, Little D dug up the bone and took it away to enjoy as his own.

As time went on, Little D had collected more bones than he could eat in a day, so he searched for his own hiding place. It took some time to find what he needed, but at last, in a cave next to a dry riverbed, he found a place that was big enough to hold many bones.

Over the next weeks and months, many bones were accumulated in the cave by Little D. Always well disguised by the red dust of the plains, he would not only stalk his brothers but his mother and father as well. Little D was stealing from his entire family!

Now all this time the sky had not filled with clouds and it had not once rained. The plains were getting drier and dustier, and dustier and drier. Little D had no trouble covering himself with his red dust disguise, and continuing on with his dishonest ways.

His cave was soon full to the top with stolen bones. Little D was so happy to know that he would not go hungry anymore. However, all his family members were by now getting quite weak. They had been robbed of their store of bones, and, with no rain for months, they were having difficulty tracking down any animals and bringing home fresh food to share with each other.

Then, one day, the weather brought a change to the land and also to Little D's dishonest ways. Rain started to fall across the plains. It started with a few drops here and there. Then, with some flashes of lightning and drums of thunder, the sky became like a wide waterfall from heaven. In fact, there was so much water falling down that the plains were soon like a silver sea, and the dry riverbed filled up and flowed over its banks.

Little D ran to higher ground as soon as the rains came. However he was not able to find any shelter up in the rocky hills and so the water washed him clean of all his red dust! Now he was once again shining white. Without his disguise he could no longer plan to stalk his brothers and get up to his dishonest tricks.

Also, with the river flowing over its banks, plenty of water filled Little D's cave of bones. The next week, after the flood had subsided, the bones were left on the floor of the cave, clean and washed. When the rain had stopped and the sun was out in full glory in the sky, there the bones sat, gleaming white inside the dark hole.

Little D returned to the cave and he saw the bones shining white and clean. When he looked at the bones – shining white and clean and then looked at his coat – shining white and clean, he knew in his heart that it was time to give the bones back to his family. That night he carried them one by one out onto the plains and scattered them over the ground.

The next morning his family found the scattered bones, gathered them up and shared them together. They never knew who had been taking them and where they had been taken to, but this didn't seem to matter. What did matter however, was that Little D was watching his family as they collected their bone treasures, and he saw how happily they were sharing together. Suddenly, seeing his family happy seemed like the best thing in the world. Had the red dust disguise stopped him from seeing this before?

Little D also discovered that he had now grown strong enough to hunt for his own food. He wasn't Little D anymore, but a handsome big Dingo! And as time went by, he was soon stalking animals for his family, and bringing home food to feed his own children. And he took care that the youngest and smallest always had enough to eat.

Anansi and the Statue

The Anansi stories originated in West Africa and were then taken to the islands of the Caribbean along with the transportation of slaves from Africa to America. They are also known as Spider Stories – 'Anansi' was both a man and a spider! Stories of Kweku Anansi are still told by the Ashanti people in Ghana. Similar stories with different heroes are told elsewhere around the world: Rabbit is the main character in the stories in the French West Indies, southern United States, and East Africa; in Nigeria, Tortoise is the mischief-maker. The Anansi / Spider stories are a wonderful resource for six- to ten-year-olds, and an interesting contrast to the Spiderman character from popular movies. As in all communities, not everyone does as she is supposed to, and this is why the character of Anansi came into being. Anansi the Spider Man is lazy, dishonest and very greedy. He is full of naughty tricks, but funny and lovable. Usually his greedy and dishonest behaviour is punished by natural consequences, and humour carries the theme to the end. Included here is an example of how Anansi's dishonesty meets just deserts.

Once upon a time, Kweku Anansi lived in a small village. The people of this village were very united. One day, the chief of the village called his people to him and suggested the idea of having a farm that would feed everyone in the village in times of famine. Every one embraced the idea except Anansi who said that he was sick. Any time the others called him to join them on the farm, he lied that he was sick.

Fridays were set aside for work on the farm. Work on the farm went very well without Anansi who always lied that he was too sick to work. But when it was almost time for harvesting, the chief and his people realised that someone had started to steal the produce. Each week when they went to the farm they realised that someone was harvesting portions of the food. News of the thefts spread very fast across the whole village. The chief summoned the village folk to work out a plan to help them catch the thief. Anansi himself was not at the meeting because he claimed he was sick.

People suggested various ways of catching the thief, but the simplest and best one was for a big statue made from quick drying glue to be placed in the middle of the farm. Anyone who touched it would get stuck to it.

The next night, Anansi went out to continue his dubious nocturnal activity. He didn't know what plans the people had taken to arrest the thief. When he arrived at the farm, he saw something like a human being in the middle of the fields.

Anansi quickly shouted, 'Who is that? Who is that? What are you doing in the farm at this time of the night?' There was no answer. Anansi continued to question the statue thinking that it was a human being. He got very close and said, 'Hey man, if you do not answer me I will slap you with my left hand.' And before he could end his statement, he had slapped the supposed human with his left hand. His left hand got stuck to the glue statue. Anansi thought that the individual was holding him and so he shouted further in anger saying: 'Look my friend; I asked you a simple question and now you have held my left hand without any provocation. Please let go my left hand else I will slap you with my right hand.' But before Anansi finished saying this, he slapped the statue again with his right hand and it also got stuck!

Anansi was now becoming furious and also quite alarmed because day was already breaking. He started to kick the statue with his legs in an attempt to free himself. Both of his legs also got stuck. Kweku Anansi was now hanging on the statue with no one to rescue him.

The next morning, the elders of the town travelled to the farm to see if luck was on their side in arresting the mysterious thief. They saw Anansi hanging on the statue. Quickly, word got to the village and everybody rushed to the farm to see Anansi hanging on the statue. It was a big shame for Kweku Anansi and his family. The villagers then set Anansi free from the statue and hooted at him. Unable to bear the shame, Anansi took to his heels and went and hid in the topmost corner of his room. This is the reason why we always find Anansi the Spider in the top corners of our rooms. Also, because of the shame, this is the reason why Anansi always shies away when he sees people approaching.

Akimba and the Magic Cow

Once upon a time there was a very poor man called Akimba. He had no money and no food. One day he went to the forest looking for something to eat. Here he met an old man cutting wood and he stopped to help him. The old man was so grateful that he gave Akimba a cow in return. He told him to go home and say to the cow, 'Coo, coo, coo'.

When Akimba arrived home he said 'Coo, coo, coo' to the cow and the cow gave him a gold coin. He kept saying 'Coo, coo, coo' until he was a wealthy man.

Then came the time when Akimba had to go away on a journey. He asked his neighbour Bumba to mind the cow, but asked him not to ever say 'Coo, coo, coo'. As soon as Akimba left, Bumba said 'Coo, coo, coo' and the cow gave him a gold coin. Bumba was very pleased with this and decided to keep the cow for himself. When Akimba returned he was given a different cow, and when Akimba said 'Coo, coo, coo' all this cow did was moo!

Akimba returned to the old man in the forest to tell him what had happened. The old man gave him a sheep and said to say 'boo, roo, roo' when he reached home. The sheep gave him a silver coin and Akimba became wealthy saying 'boo, roo, roo'. Eventually he had to go on another trip and he left the sheep with his neighbour with the warning not to say 'boo, roo, roo'. Bumba soon found out that the sheep gave silver coins, and on Akimba's return he kept the magic sheep and gave him another one in its place. All that the new sheep would do when Akimba said 'boo, roo, roo' was say 'baa, baa, baa'!

As before, Akimba returned to the old man in the forest and this time was given a chicken and told to say 'cluck, cluck, cluck'. When Akimba reached home he said 'cluck, cluck, cluck' and the chicken laid an egg. 'Eggs are eggs' Akimba said and since he was hungry he ate the egg. Then he sold many more eggs and eventually became a wealthy man again. Soon he had to go on another journey and left the chicken with his neighbour Bumba and told him not to ever say 'cluck, cluck, cluck'. As before, Bumba swapped the chicken with another chicken that would not lay an egg when Akimba said 'cluck, cluck, cluck'.

This time Akimba carried the chicken back to the forest. The old man gave him a stick to take home and told him to say 'stick dance for me' and then to say 'Mamba' to make it stop. Once back inside his hut Akimba said 'stick dance for me' and the stick began to beat him until he remembered to say 'Mamba'. Akimba had started to suspect his neighbour Bamba and so he pretended he had to go away on another trip. He asked Bamba to mind the stick and not to say 'stick dance for me'. Of course, as soon as Akimba was around the first corner of the path, Bumba called out 'stick dance for me'. The stick began to beat him and Akimba heard his cries from along the path. He came back and Bamba agreed to return the cow, the sheep and the chicken if Akimba could stop the beating stick. Akimba cried out 'Mamba' and the stick stopped. He took his animals home and was never hungry or poor again.

Cherry Red

I wrote this little story for a five-year-old girl who displayed sneaky behaviour when visiting a friend's home. My friend had a gnome statue in her garden. Although the little girl knew the statue was quite old and should not be touched, she would wait till no one was looking and sit out in the garden trying to peel off its red paint. Instead of addressing negative behaviour, the story tries to bring a positive message to the little girl about how much the gnome liked the colour red. The effect of the story was immediate – the child stopped peeling off the paint.

There was once a little gnome who lived with his brothers and sisters under the roots of a great fig tree. This tree was in the middle of an old rainforest, near a long beach by the sea.

The little gnome loved to wander and gather beautiful things to bring back to show his family. Most of all he loved anything that was the colour red. His mother had knitted him a bright red cap, and soon he was known to all his forest friends as Cherry Red.

Whenever Cherry Red had time to spare, he would wander here and there through the forest, collecting red-tipped leaves, red berries and other red kinds of forest things.

As time went on, he found himself wandering further and further along the paths, until he came one day to the edge of the forest and found a little garden at the back of a red brick house.

Cherry Red could not believe his eyes when he entered the garden – never before had he seen so many beautiful flowers and fruits in one place. He was sure there were many more red things here than in his entire forest! There were red geraniums, red roses and red bottlebrush. Growing up and along the fence, there was a giant tomato vine, all covered with cherry red tomatoes. And in the vegetable patch there were shiny red strawberries poking their little heads out between the green strawberry leaves.

Cherry Red was so happy! He picked two little tomatoes and one strawberry (being very careful to leave enough for the folk who owned the garden) and he ran all the way back along the forest path to show his family.

All the way home he was so happy that he made up a little song and sang to himself:

> *Cherry Red is a happy fellow,*
> *In hat of red and coat of yellow,*
> *Gathering treasures from the garden today,*
> *Zippity dippity dippity zay!*

And do you know, from that day to this, Cherry Red has returned to this special garden every morning. He sits there all day to look out over his red treasures – the tomatoes, the strawberries and the flowers – and every evening he returns to the forest taking a small red gift back to his family.

i   Stealing in younger children, however, is often not 'stealing' at all, but just imitation of adults 'owning' things. In older children it can sometimes be a symptom of disturbance related to a need for more attention, rather than just 'bad' behaviour. As we have seen, a therapeutic story needs to be combined with enquiry into the child's home circumstances.

11

Disrespectful or Uncaring

Tembe's Boots

This simple story was written for an Educare Centre in Cape Town to help children learn to put their shoes together. Refer to Chapter Three for more detail on its use and effect. It has universal value and can be used with children three years and upwards.

Tembe was a little boy who came each day to kindergarten just like you. Every morning when he woke up he would get dressed and put on his favourite red boots that he liked to wear to school.

Tembe's red boots were the most favourite thing that he liked to wear. He would sit eating breakfast and sometimes take a peep under the table – yes, there his red boots were waiting – on his feet, on the floor under the table, so happy to be side by side, so happy to be 'friends together'.

If he listened very carefully, he could hear them softly singing:

Friends together, diddley-deather, we're so happy to be 'friends together'.

On the way to school, whenever Tembe walked, his boots walked too. Whenever Tembe jumped, his boots jumped too. Whenever Tembe hopped, his boots hopped too. He would often look down at them and smile – he could see how much they liked to be 'friends together'.

When he was playing in the garden at school he would sometimes sit on the swing and look down at his boots and click them together – how happy they were to be on his feet and be 'friends together'.

Listen – can you hear them sing:

Friends together, diddley-deather, we're so happy to be 'friends together'.

Then came a time each day when his teacher would call the children onto the veranda – it was time to come in for a sleep. Tembe had to take off his red boots and leave them outside – of course, his boots couldn't come inside for rest time! Carefully he placed them against the wall, to wait for him – 'friends together'. There they would sit until rest time was finished and it was time to put them back on his feet for the long walk home.

Tembe would lie on his bed in the schoolroom and listen to his teacher singing lullabies. And when his teacher stopped singing, just as he was falling asleep, he could softly, ever so softly, hear his boots on the veranda singing:

Friends together, diddley-deather, we're so happy to be 'friends together'.

The Pocket Knife and the Castle

A story written for an eight-year-old boy who was being irresponsible with tools. I have also used this story in schools and vacation care programs to encourage older children to create things with their hands – in wood or clay or soapstone. I use a special prop in telling this – a small wooden log carved like a jigsaw puzzle – this can be shaken out into a simple castle shape at the point in the story when the boy's family wakes up and finds what he has made. An improvised, roughly-carved or clay-moulded castle would do just as well.

There was once a young boy who had been given a pocket-knife for his birthday. A brand new pocket-knife, a gleaming shining pocket-knife. A very sharp pocket-knife, that itched to be used.

He kept it in his pocket – and there it stayed, itching to be used.

I am a knife and I love to cut; open me, use me, then shut me back up.

The boy was sure he could hear it singing to him sometimes. But what could a boy use a pocket-knife for?

I am a knife and I love to cut; open me, use me, then shut me back up.

There, he could hear it again. He was sitting in the kitchen, and nobody was around. He pulled out his knife and started to cut away at the table leg. The knife was so happy to be used – but when his mother came into the kitchen she was not happy! She took the pocket-knife away for a month and a day.

Finally it was back in the boy's pocket, itching to be used.

I am a knife and I love to cut; open me, use me, then shut me back up.

The boy could hear it singing to him again. He was in the lounge room, and nobody was around. He pulled out his knife and started to cut into the cushion on grandmother's chair. The knife was so happy to be used – but when his grandmother came into the lounge room she was not happy! She took the pocket-knife away for a month and a day.

Finally it was back in the boy's pocket, itching to be used.

I am a knife and I love to cut; open me, use me, then shut me back up.

The boy could hear it singing to him again. He was in the shed, and nobody was around. He pulled out his knife and started to cut notches into the workbench. The knife was so happy to be used – but when his grandfather came into his shed he was not happy! He took the pocket-knife away for a month and a day.

Finally it was back in the boy's pocket, once again itching to be used.

That night the boy fell asleep in the silver light of the moon shining down through his bedroom window. While in a deep sleep, the boy had a dream. In this dream there was a hill and on this hill there was a castle and in this castle there were some windows and behind the windows there were many rooms and in these rooms there were some ...

At this point the boy woke up, sat up in bed and had a wonderful idea. 'I know what to do with my pocket-knife' he said. He climbed out of bed, dressed himself, and put his pocket-knife into his pocket. Then he went out into the garden and in the light of the moon found a small log lying down near the compost heap.

[Show the listeners a small log]

He brought the log onto the veranda, opened up his pocket-knife, and by the silver light of the moon he set to work. And all the while he was working, the pocket-knife was singing:

I am a knife and I love to cut; open me, use me, then shut me back up.

And all the while he was working the rest of his family was still fast asleep.

[Ask listeners to close their eyes for one minute]

When they woke up, there on the kitchen table was a beautiful surprise.

[Show the listeners a carved, wooden castle]

On the lounge was the young boy, fast asleep. And in his pocket was a very happy, but very tired pocket-knife!

From that day on, whenever the boy looked through the windows of his wooden castle, he always had a new idea for how to use his pocket-knife. His pocket-knife was always happy, and so was the boy's family. This young boy grew up to be a wood carver, famous for the castles he could carve out of a simple piece of wood.

Ball of Wool Poem

A poem can sometimes touch the imagination as deeply as a story. A parent at a Creative Discipline workshop used the following to deal with the challenge of her four-year-old daughter wanting to use scissors to chop things to pieces. Of course, cutting with scissors is a natural skill to master for a four-year-old, but the mother was having difficulty keeping the 'cutting' in check. She wrote the 'Ball of Wool' to coincide with a $100 order of wool that had arrived for her craft workshops – the poem was tucked into the wool-bag and she pulled it out, feigned surprise at its presence, and then read it out to her daughter. The little girl was so taken by the message that she promptly took her doll out of its cradle and tucked some of the woollen balls into bed. She treated them like babies for the next few days. Cutting into the balls with scissors was never an issue.

A Ball of Wool by Jane Dolahenty

A ball of wool brings hours of joy to all who take the time –
Of picking out a treasured ball and learning tricks of mine.

Knit me, weave me, make a doll – Oh, the things we can create,
But being cut in tiny bits … there is no worse a fate!

Scissors really frighten me, please keep me safe at bay,
I'm happiest just right near you, as you work away.

And please don't let me roll around, all loosely on the floor,
I may get kicked or trodden on, and tangled up for sure.

And when you have all finished with me, and cut your length of thread,
Please roll me up all snug and neat and place me in my bed.

Instructions: Please find a special bed for your new family of wool!

The Little Girl Who Loved Flowers

A story written for a four-year-old girl who had recently moved out of the Nairobi slums to a boarding school in the country. This little girl had never seen flowers growing in gardens before and she delighted in continually picking them. Meanwhile the housemother was getting very upset about this, as was the school gardener. The story was written in an attempt to redirect the girl's behaviour, and was successful. The house-mother helped by providing some coloured pieces of wool for the rainbow dancing stick.

There was once a little girl called Netty who lived with her mother and many, many brothers and sisters. Little Netty loved flowers. She loved the patterns of flowers, the shapes of flowers, the smell of flowers... but most of all she loved the beautiful colours of flowers ...red, pink, purple, yellow, orange, blue... so many wonderful colours.

Little Netty would spend all her spare time wandering the garden and looking for flowers to pick and play with. She would collect them all and spread them on the grass. Then she would sit amongst them, pulling off the petals and playing with them and throwing them up in the air.

One day while little Netty was sitting in the grass, playing with some yellow nasturtium petals, she heard a whispering on the breeze. It sounded as if it was coming from a green daisy bush nearby. Little Netty moved closer, and right inside the daisy bush she saw a tiny bud opening and closing. It seemed to be talking to her!

'Please don't pick my sisters and brothers all the time, little girl. Once we have been taken from our green bushes we fade and die. But if you leave us growing then we can keep on dancing in the garden. There is nothing a flower likes to do more than dance'.

Little Netty didn't know what to say! She also loved to dance so she perfectly understood what the flower bud was saying.

Then she had an idea. She went to her mother and asked her for a piece of wool for every colour of her favourite flowers. Then she tied all the brightly coloured pieces to a long stick and went outside. With her rainbow stick held high she started to dance across the grass and around the garden.

Soon the breeze joined in, gently blowing the flowers backwards and forwards, and all together they danced with little Netty in the garden.

The tiny new daisy bud was very happy to see this, and she smiled such a big smile that all her white daisy petals popped out and spread open. Then she too joined with little Netty in the dance.

Grandmother and the Donkey

A story to encourage litter awareness.

This story was written in 1997 for a puppet show for African children, then toured through kindergartens in the Cape Town townships. The effect was immediate – as the puppeteers were packing up the show, the children would be running up to them with handfuls of litter. I believe the story has a universal message and could be used with all ages. The Xhosa song was written by one of the puppeteers, Maria Msebenzi.

Once upon a time, in the southern lands of Africa, there lived an old grandmother. Her children and grandchildren had moved into the town and she was left by herself on her farm in the country. But grandmother never felt lonely because her favourite child was 'nature' itself, and there was always so much to do to take care of nature.

Grandmother especially liked to see her nature child wearing a beautiful dress, a flower dress, and so she spent most of her time tending a garden and growing beautiful flowers. Her best friend and helper was a little brown donkey who worked all day pulling a cart to carry buckets of water for the flower garden. Then on Saturdays he would carry Grandmother on his strong back, pulling a cartload of flowers behind him, and set off for the market at the edge of town. Grandmother would dress him up for the day with a special hat ringed with flowers and a brightly coloured cloth on his back.

At the end of the day, when all the flowers had been sold, Grandmother would use the money to buy food for herself and oats for the little brown donkey. They always had enough to eat, and for a long time they were very happy working and living together. The donkey loved Grandmother and Grandmother loved the donkey. As they worked together in the flower garden she would often sing this song to him:

> *Oh, a donkey is a wonderful thing; a wonderful thing is a donkey.*
> *Imbongolo yinto entle kahle; into ekahle yimbongolo.*

However, as the years went by, Grandmother grew older and older, and there came a time when she was too old to work in her flower garden and too old to live out in the country by herself. So one day she packed all her belongings into the donkey cart, put the flower hat on the donkey's head and the brightly coloured cloth on his back, and together they set off to town to find a new house, a town house, to live in.

Now Grandmother had not been into town for a very long time, and as she travelled up and down the streets on the way to her new house, she was shocked and saddened to find what an untidy place it had become. There was mess and garbage piled up everywhere. Instead of gardens of flowers there were gardens of mess and garbage.

'What are the people doing to 'nature's child', cried Grandmother. 'How can they dress her in such an ugly dress?' And she sat down amongst the tins and bottles and plastic bags outside her new house and started to cry. While she was crying the little brown donkey came close to her and bent down and whispered a secret in her ear. Slowly Grandmother's tears stopped and a smile crept across her wrinkled old face. 'Of course, little brown donkey, what a wonderful idea' she said, and then she started to sing:

> *Oh, a donkey is a wonderful thing; a wonderful thing is a donkey.*
> *Imbongolo yinto entle kahle; into ekahle yimbongolo.*

While she was singing she unpacked all her belongings into her new house. After a cup of tea for herself and some water and oats for the donkey, she then set off down the street with the donkey and an empty cart. As she walked she started to pick up the garbage and load it onto the cart. And as she worked she sang:

My nature's child is ugly and grey, She needs a change of dress today.
Let's pick up the garbage and clean up the mess,
Then plant seeds to grow a flower dress.

It wasn't long before the children in the street heard Grandmother's happy singing. They came out of their houses and started to help. By the end of the first day, with the children working hard, all the garbage in the first street had been picked up. It was loaded onto the donkey cart and taken to the garbage tip. Then Grandmother dipped her hand into a bag of flower seeds that she had brought from her country garden, and gave seeds to all the children to take back home and plant in front of their houses.

The next day, with more children helping, the second street was cleaned up. The next day, the third street was tidied. In this way, with the children working with Grandmother and the little brown donkey, every street in the town was soon cleared of all the mess. And with the flower seeds planted in front of all the houses, soon 'nature's child' had a new town dress, a beautiful flower dress.

Grandmother was now able to enjoy the beauty of the flowers in the town. Meanwhile the little brown donkey was kept busy carrying water up and down the streets for all the gardens, and also collecting new garbage every day.

From that day to this, if anyone in the town had any garbage to throw out, they would put it in their bins and wait until the donkey cart came by to load it for the tip. Each day the children would pick flowers from their garden and weave a fresh flower ring for the donkey's hat.

If you ever visit this town you will hear the people singing praises to the little brown donkey – the little brown donkey who helped Grandmother give their town a beautiful new dress, a flower dress:

Oh, a donkey is a wonderful thing; a wonderful thing is a donkey.
Imbongolo yinto entle kahle; into ekahle yimbongolo.

The Old Woman and the Ants

This is a delightful story that I first heard in an Educare playgroup in Cape Town. It was from an anonymous source and has been re-written for this book. It was being told as a puppet show to three-year-olds. It has a simple message for all ages about taking care of the smallest details in life!

There was once an old woman who always left the top off her sugar jar. Every day when she was taking tea, she spooned the sugar into her cup and then left the sugar jar open on the cupboard.

This old woman had a pet tortoise who lived in her house. The tortoise often said, 'Take care, old woman, or the ants will come one day and steal your sugar!'

But the old woman just laughed and carried on drinking her tea.

The days and weeks went by, and then one day the tortoise's prediction came to pass.

The ants, that normally kept politely to themselves out in the garden, came into the kitchen, up onto the cupboard and into the sugar jar. Grain by grain they started to carry off the sugar.

The next day, when the old woman was making her tea, she put her spoon into the sugar jar and was surprised to find that not one grain of sugar was left.

The tortoise was tempted to say, 'I told you so', but he was too wise for such comments. Instead he told the old woman that he had watched the ants taking the sugar and knew where their hiding place was. The woman followed the tortoise to a little hole under the steps, and sure enough, when she looked inside, there was a pile of sugar grains.

The old woman was able to reach in with her spoon and get just enough sugar for one cup of tea.

Later that day she took some coins from her drawer and walked to the shop to buy a new bag of sugar. As soon as she reached home, she went straight to the kitchen and poured the sugar into the jar.

Then, do you know what the old woman did? She screwed the lid tightly onto the jar and never again did she lose her sugar to the ants. The ants stayed in the garden and the sugar stayed in the jar.

12

Greedy or Unable to Share

Garden of Light – an environmental fairytale

Garden of Light was written for World Environment Day in 1992 and later produced as a one-hour musical play by Home Grown Productions, Byron Bay. Refer to Chapter Three for details on the uses and effects of this story. Suitable for age 6 and upwards.

There was once a beautiful garden that stretched far and wide, from the valleys to the plains, from the hills to the seaside.

In this beautiful garden grew every flower, every plant, every tree. In this beautiful garden lived every bird, every butterfly, every bee.

In this beautiful garden all the children of the land loved to play, and the garden kept them healthy and happy in their play everyday.

In the centre of this garden, at the top of the tallest hill, was a great shining golden ball. The golden ball shone so bright, it filled the garden with springtime light.

At the foot of the hill lived the caretaker of the golden ball. She was a Nature Weaver and it was her task to polish the ball and keep it shining bright. She lived in a room with a round weaving basket and a weaving loom.

Every day she would take her round basket into the garden and fill it with fresh grasses and flowers and leaves. Then on her weaving loom she would weave a soft nature cloth.

With this soft nature cloth she would climb to the top of the hill and polish the golden ball so bright – until it filled the garden with glorious springtime light.

For a long time all was happy and well. The golden ball needed the garden and the garden needed the golden ball. And the children enjoyed somewhere beautiful to play.

*

But one day a new King took over the land. This new King was called King-Didn't-Care and King-Didn't-Care didn't care about anything except himself. King-Didn't-Care didn't care about flowers and plants and trees. King-Didn't-Care didn't care about birds and butterflies and bees. King-Didn't-Care didn't care if the children had anywhere beautiful to play.

King-Didn't-Care only cared about what *he* liked, and King-Didn't-Care only liked collecting and storing treasures. So as soon as King-Didn't-Care took over the land he ordered his workmen to start digging treasure mines and building castles to store treasures in.

And slowly, very slowly, the beautiful garden was chopped down to make way for treasure mines and treasure castles.

*

As the garden grew smaller and smaller, the Nature Weaver found it harder and harder to fill her round basket with fresh flowers and grasses and leaves. She found it harder and harder to weave a soft nature cloth on her weaving loom. She found it harder and harder to polish the golden ball bright, and slowly the golden ball stopped shining its glorious springtime light. Slowly the golden ball started to turn a tarnished grey, the grey of the clouds on a dark stormy day.

Soon, all the beautiful garden was gone. There were no more flowers and plants and trees, there were no more birds and butterflies and bees. And there was nowhere beautiful for the children to play.

All that was left at the top of the tallest hill was a great grey tarnished ball. In the room at the foot of the hill sat the Nature Weaver with an empty weaving basket and an empty weaving loom. The land around was now barren and brown. It was filled with holes where treasure mines had been dug, and covered with castles to store treasures in.

*

Many years passed. The garden was forgotten and the children grew used to having nowhere beautiful to play. King-Didn't-Care didn't care that the beautiful garden was gone. He visited his castles and was kept happy counting his treasures. But one day he happened to look out of a castle window and see the hill of the grey tarnished ball.

'What a terrible sight', he said to himself. 'This grey tarnished ball I must try to hide – it makes me feel sort of uncomfortable inside'.

King-Didn't-Care then ordered his workmen to build a high stone wall around the hill of the grey tarnished ball. The high stone wall had no windows and no doors. No one could get in to see the grey tarnished ball, and the Nature Weaver couldn't get out. She stayed sitting in her room, with her empty weaving basket and her empty weaving loom.

*

On the morning after the wall was finished King-Didn't-Care woke up feeling quite ill. When he looked in his mirror he saw that he had turned quite grey, the grey of the clouds on a dark stormy day. The doctors in the land were called to his bedside. They had never seen such an illness before, and no matter what remedy they tried, nothing seemed to help. In fact, King-Didn't-Care was growing greyer by the day, and his illness became so severe that he didn't survive to see the springtime of that year.

*

On the day that King-Didn't-Care died, cracks started to appear in the high stone wall. These cracks in the wall were very small, but playing just near the wall was a child, also very small. The child found that she was able to fit through one of the cracks, and once inside she stood looking up at the hill and the great grey tarnished ball. She then saw the room at the foot of the hill, and walked up to it and peered inside. Sitting in the room was the Nature Weaver with her empty weaving basket and empty weaving loom.

The Nature Weaver smiled a tired but friendly smile. 'I hope you've come in time' she said. Beckoning the little child to come inside, she told the story of the beautiful garden that once stretched over the land; of the flowers and plants and trees; of the birds and butterflies and bees. She told of her basket that she used to fill with fresh flowers and grasses and leaves. She told of her weaving loom and the soft nature cloth she used to weave. She told of her task to polish the golden ball and keep it shining bright, so that it would fill the garden with springtime light.

The little child's eyes grew wide with wonder. 'We must bring back the garden and we must bring back the golden shine to the great grey tarnished ball' she cried.

'Well', the Nature Weaver sighed, 'there is a way to do this but I am too old to do it by myself. I would need your help and the help of all the other children in the land. You must be prepared to work very hard. Go back through a crack in the wall and gather up all the children you can find – then I will tell you what we need to do. I hope you've come in time, I do hope you've come in time!'

*

The little child slipped back out through a crack in the wall and gathered up as many children as she could find. They followed her back to the Nature Weaver's room where they all sat down to watch and listen. The Nature Weaver took out a small box and held it for the children to see. 'These are my treasures,' she said, 'I gathered them from the garden before it was chopped down'. Then she opened the lid of the box and the children saw thousands of tiny seeds inside. 'With your help and much hard work we can plant these seeds and bring back the garden. Then I will be able to weave a new nature cloth and with this cloth we may be able to bring back the shine to the grey tarnished ball.'

The Nature Weaver showed the children how to dig the ground and plant the seeds, and how to water and tend the new plants with loving care. Every day the children would come back through the cracks in the wall and work in the garden at the foot of the hill of the grey tarnished ball.

When the garden had grown high enough the Nature Weaver gave the children her round weaving basket to fill with fresh grasses and flowers and leaves. She then sat at her weaving loom and once more she was able to weave a soft nature cloth. The children then took the soft nature cloth to the top of the hill and started to polish the grey tarnished ball. This took a very long time – for many days the children came back through the crack in the wall and polished and polished the grey tarnished ball.

And slowly, slowly, slowly (it took a very long time) the children were able to bring back the golden shine. The great ball once again started to shine so bright, it filled the garden at the foot of the hill with golden springtime light. The children kept polishing and polishing the golden ball, until one day its golden light shone so brightly against the high stone wall that it caused the high stone wall … to fall!

The golden light then flooded out over the land, and the beautiful garden was once more able to stretch far and wide, from the valleys to the plains, from the hills to the seaside. And once more, as before, the children had somewhere beautiful to play.

Greedy Possum

I wrote this story with several aims in mind. It is not a story for three- or four-year-olds – at this young age greed is not a conscious reality! However, in our modern world this story could be quite useful for children aged five or more who want everything and are continually influenced by commercial messages in the media. It is a quite a long story, and highlights the bountiful treasures of nature.

Little possum was not born greedy. She was just born with a love of beautiful things, especially things that shimmered and sparkled and shone. While her mother was teaching her how to find the best fruits and seeds to eat, little possum was looking elsewhere, watching how the silver moonlight shimmered on the dancing leaves.

While her mother was showing her how to look for safe homes high up in hollow trees, little possum was busy looking up in wonderment at all the sparkling stars in the night sky.

While her mother was telling her about the dangers to be aware of in the bushland, little possum was counting all the shiny colours in the early morning dewdrops.

*

Then something happened that changed little possum's life forever!

Early one morning, when the birds were just waking up and the night animals – like possums – were on their way home to sleep, little possum came across a nest in the grass full of things that shimmered and sparkled and shone. Excited about her discovery, she bent down and reached out to touch the wonderful treasures. There were blue beads of shimmering glass, sparkling marble balls and shiny bottle tops. Little possum had never before been close to such beautiful things – treasures she could actually touch and hold in her possum paws.

Suddenly a dark blue bird flew down from the branch above.

'What are you doing with *my* treasures', squawked the bowerbird and he started to peck and poke at little possum's head.

'I was just touching – they are so beautiful' called back little possum as she ran off into the bush to escape the treasures' angry owner.

She hid herself under a thick leafy branch, well out of harm's way. For the rest of the morning, while her possum family was fast asleep, she looked out at the special treasures in the bowerbird's nest and wished she could have some for herself.

You see, little possum had learnt something new this day – she had learnt that beautiful things could actually belong to someone. 'This is much better than the treasures in the bushland that can just be looked at', thought little possum longingly.

*

From that day on, all that little possum could think about was how she could find some treasures of her own. She started to search far and wide for things that shimmered and sparkled and shone – just like the ones she had seen in the bowerbird's nest. She searched through the bushland valleys. She searched over the bushland hills. She wandered far and wide, until finally she reached the open fields – exactly where her mother had told her never to go.

'That's where the *humans* live', her mother had warned. And sure enough, out in the wide clearing little possum saw many two-legged *humans* – tall and short and fat and thin. She also saw many large wooden houses with beautiful gardens all around.

It was above one of these gardens that little possum saw the bowerbird flying away with a string of shiny blue beads in his beak.

Little possum was so excited. If the bowerbird was collecting treasures from the *humans'* gardens, then perhaps at last she had found the place where shimmering, sparkling, shining things came from.

She couldn't wait to go exploring for her own treasures. However, something her mother had taught her jumped into her possum mind – 'Wait until night-time, possums are much safer at night than during the day'.

So she curled up in the branch of a tree at the edge of the open fields and waited until it was dark enough to go exploring. And this night was the beginning of little possum turning into *greedy possum!*

*

Every garden that she dared to enter led her to something that shimmered or sparkled or shone. Lying on the grass or under bushes she found shimmering pieces of glass, sparkling marbles, and shiny coins. On the pathways and in the gardens she found shimmering beads, sparkling spoons, and shiny keys. Greedy possum crept around the houses while all the *humans* were fast asleep and gathered up as many treasures as she could carry.

And where does a greedy possum carry treasures you may wonder? In her possum pouch of course! And the more treasures that greedy possum stuffed into her pouch, the bigger she grew and the heavier she became and the slower she moved.

By the time she had finished exploring all the human gardens, greedy possum was so big and heavy that it took all her strength to cross the open fields and reach the shelter of her bushland home. As the sun rose the next morning, greedy possum was safely curled up inside a hollow log, deep in the bush.

Greedy possum was very happy. But greedy possum was also very tired, and soon she fell into a deep sleep. All day she slept, and the next night, and the next day.

Finally she woke up, feeling very hungry. But how does a possum with a possum pouch full of heavy treasures go hunting for food?

Just then, greedy possum heard a familiar noise and smelt a familiar smell. She looked out and saw her mother coming along the ground towards her. 'Little possum, I have been so worried about you. What have you been doing?' she cried.

'I have been collecting many treasures' said greedy possum, and she opened the possum pouch for her mother to peep inside.

Mother possum shook her head. 'Dear little possum, we don't need *human* treasures to make us happy. Your possum pouch needs to be saved for a more special treasure than things that shimmer or sparkle or shine.'

Mother possum then offered to help take everything out of little possum's pouch so that they could go hunting together. She knew little possum must be very hungry.

But greedy possum did not want to listen to her mother, and definitely did not want to give up her treasures. 'No,' she cried, 'these treasures are mine, all mine', and she moved further back inside the log and curled up into a tight ball. For a long time she stayed like this till her mother lost interest in waiting and continued on her hunt to look for fruits and seeds to eat.

*

Some time later, greedy possum heard scampering and many possum noises. When she looked up she saw many of her possum friends waiting outside the hollow log. News of her visit to the 'human' gardens had travelled fast through the bushland. Her friends had come to see what she had found.

Greedy possum opened her pouch for them to have a peep at her collection of treasures. Of course, when the other possums saw all the things that shimmered and sparkled and shone, they wanted to have some of their own. But greedy possum did not want to share!

'No,' cried greedy possum, 'these treasures are mine, all mine', and she moved further back inside the log and curled up once again into a tight ball. For a long time she stayed like this till her friends lost interest in waiting and continued on their hunt to look for fruits and seeds to eat.

*

Greedy possum slept and slept – what else was there to do? She was too heavy to go hunting for food, and she didn't dare take her treasures out of her pouch and leave them behind. Someone might come and take them.

So greedy possum grew more and more hungry. And more and more lonely. Her mother did not return. Her friends did not return. She sat inside her hollow log and looked out at the world and realised that even with all her new treasures she was not a happy possum.

Then, early one morning, through her teary big brown eyes, she saw a dewdrop shining with colours in the wet grass outside. It reminded her of the time when she used to be happy enjoying the natural treasures of the bushland.

'What a silly possum I have been,' she cried to herself, 'it is time to empty my pouch and be free of these heavy things.' She crawled out of her hollow log and dragged herself through the bushland to where the bowerbird had his nest in the grass.

Bowerbird was very surprised to have a visitor! He watched with glee as the possum carefully lifted all the treasures out of her possum pouch and spread them on the ground. Out came the shimmering pieces of glass, sparkling marbles, and shiny coins. Out came the shimmering beads, sparkling spoons, and shiny keys. Out came all the treasures, until her possum pouch was empty and the grass was covered with things that shimmered and sparkled and shone.

Bowerbird then spent all day choosing the best things – mostly blue of course – to take into his nest. And that night wombat found the remaining treasures and took them underground to brighten up his dark earth home.

Meanwhile, possum (who was not a *greedy* nor a *little* possum anymore) scampered off to hunt for food, so happy to be light and free once again.

*

After possum had found many fruits and seeds to eat, she set to work finding a new home for herself, safe and high in a hollow tree. Then she visited her mother to show that she was not laden down anymore by a pouch full of *human* treasures. She also wanted to tell her mother that she was now big enough to live in the bushland by herself.

Not long after this, just as her mother had promised, possum found something growing in her pouch that was a much more special treasure than things that shimmered and sparkled and shone.

It was a new baby possum!

As baby possum grew and started to venture out of the possum pouch to explore the bushland, new mother possum shared with her baby her love of beautiful bushland things. Together they watched how the silver moonlight shimmered on the dancing leaves, they looked at the sparkling stars in the night sky, and they found shiny colours in early morning dewdrops.

New mother possum also taught her baby how to find the best fruits and leaves to eat, the dangers to be aware of in the bushland, and how to build a home safe and high in a hollow tree. Most importantly, new mother possum taught her baby possum to stay in the bushland and keep away from 'human' gardens, especially *human* treasures that shimmered and sparkled and shone.

The Magic Fish

Suitable for age six and older, this story is my own version of a well loved Grimm's fairytale. Also known as 'The Fisherman and his Wife', this consequential story is recommended for parents and teachers to use when their children seem never to be satisfied. A strong memory from this story is when one of my own boys, aged six, leant back in his chair after hearing it and sighed a very satisfied sigh, 'Yes, that's very fair – no one deserves to have that much!' I have added a song to the story, and because it was a favourite of the Kenyan women when I worked in East Africa, I include the words of the song in Kiswahili.

There was once a fisherman who lived with his wife in a little hut on the beach at the edge of a lagoon. He and his wife were so poor they had no money to buy any food. However they always had plenty to eat. They lived on the coconuts found on the beach and the fish from the sea. Each day the fisherman would climb into his wooden boat and sing to the wind:

Wind, sail my boat, carry me across the water, wind sail my boat.
Upepo, una endesha mashua yangu, nibebe univukishe maji,
Upepo, una endesha mashua yangu.

The wind would blow into the sails and the boat would move across the blue waters of the lagoon and out onto the great ocean. As he sailed in his boat the fisherman hoped that he would catch at least one fish for dinner that night.

One day, while his boat was rocking on the waves in the middle of the sea, a large fish took the end of his line. The fisherman pulled and pulled and pulled. Suddenly, up and over the edge of the boat and onto the wooden floor, with a large plop and a splash, landed a beautiful shiny fish – the largest fish that the fisherman had ever caught in his whole life. 'This will last for many dinners' said the fisherman as he bent down to pick up the fish and put it in his bag.

Then he stopped still and listened – it seemed that someone was talking to him. But he was alone in his boat in the middle of the great sea. The talking started again, and to his surprise he looked down and saw that it was coming from the fish itself.

Fisherman, fisherman, listen to me, I have a secret from the sea,
If you throw me back in the blue, I'll grant a magic wish for you.

The fisherman carefully picked up the fish and threw it back in the water. He then sailed his boat home across the sea to where his wife was waiting for him on the beach. He excitedly told her about what had happened, and she straight away said, 'What are we waiting for, let us wish for a better place to live, let us wish for a bigger house'.

The moment she had spoken these words their little one-roomed hut turned into a bigger and grander house, with separate rooms, and a kitchen with cupboards full of food to eat.

For many days the fisherman didn't need to go out fishing, but finally the food cupboards were empty. It was time to climb into his wooden boat and set sail across the blue waters of the lagoon and out onto the great ocean. As the boat moved across the water he started to sing to the wind:

Wind, sail my boat, carry me across the water, wind sail my boat.
Upepo, una endesha mashua yangu, nibebe univukishe maji,
Upepo, una endesha mashua yangu.

While his boat was rocking on the waves in the middle of the sea, a large fish took the end of his line. The fisherman pulled and pulled and pulled. Suddenly, up and over the edge of the boat and onto the wooden floor, with a large plop and a splash, landed a beautiful shiny fish – the same magic fish that he had caught before.

Fisherman, fisherman, listen to me, I have a secret from the sea,
If you throw me back in the blue, I'll grant a magic wish for you.

The fisherman carefully picked up the fish and threw it back in the water. He then sailed his boat home across the sea to where his wife was waiting for him on the beach. He excitedly told her about what had happened, and she straight away said, 'What are we waiting for? I am tired of living in this house, let us wish for a better place to live, let us wish for a grand palace.'

Immediately she had spoken these words their house turned into a grand palace, with many, many rooms, upstairs and downstairs, and shiny towers. The palace also had gardens with many flowers and water fountains, and an even bigger kitchen with cupboards full of food to eat.

For many, many weeks to follow, the fisherman didn't need to go out fishing. But finally the food cupboards were empty. It was time to climb into his wooden boat and set sail across the blue waters of the lagoon and out onto the great ocean. As the boat moved across the water he started to sing to the wind:

> *Wind, sail my boat, carry me across the water, wind sail my boat.*
> *Upepo, una endesha mashua yangu, nibebe univukishe maji,*
> *Upepo, una endesha mashua yangu.*

While his boat was rocking on the waves in the middle of the sea, a large fish took the end of his line. The fisherman pulled and pulled and pulled. Suddenly, up and over the edge of the boat and onto the wooden floor, with a large plop and a splash, landed a beautiful shiny fish – the same magic fish that he had caught before.

> *Fisherman, fisherman, listen to me, I have a secret from the sea,*
> *If you throw me back in the blue, I'll grant a magic wish for you.*

The fisherman carefully picked up the fish and threw it back in the water. He then sailed his boat home across the sea to where his wife was waiting for him on the beach. He excitedly told her about what had happened, and she straight away said, 'What are we waiting for? I am tired of just owning a palace, let us wish for more, let us wish to own everything in the world, even the moon and the sun.'

This time the fisherman knew that his wife was expecting much more than her fair share, but it was too late to stop the wish, as the words had already been spoken. And to their surprise, in front of their very eyes, something different happened. The palace disappeared and all that was left on the beach was the little hut they had always lived in.

From this time onwards, the only food they had to eat was the coconuts found on the beach and the fish from the sea. Every day the fisherman would climb into his wooden boat and set sail across the blue waters of the lagoon and out onto the great ocean. As the boat moved across the water he would sing to the wind:

Wind, sail my boat, carry me across the water, wind sail my boat.
Upepo, una endesha mashua yangu, nibebe univukishe maji,
Upepo, una endesha mashua yangu.

For the rest of his days, the fisherman never saw the magic fish again, but he and his wife never wanted for food to eat. The sea always provided them with plenty of fish and the beach always provided them with plenty of coconuts.

'Greedy' Anansi stories

The Anansi stories originated in West Africa and then were taken to the islands of the Caribbean (see Chapter Ten).

Anansi the Spider Man is lazy, dishonest and very, very greedy. He is full of naughty tricks, but funny and lovable. Included here, for seven years and older, are three examples of how Anansi's greed meets its just deserts.

Anansi and his Shadow

Once upon a time, there lived a greedy spider called Kwaku Anansi. Such was his greed that he did not care about his wife and children, he thought only of himself. It was always Anansi, Anansi, Anansi – everything for himself.

One day Kwaku Anansi saw three ripe mangoes on a tree by the river. His mouth started watering and he yearned so much for the mangoes that he decided to go and pick them at once. He climbed the tree and soon reached the top. He plucked the first and second mango and was going to the third when he looked down into the water and saw his reflection. Thinking it was another person with some more mangoes, he felt very envious. He wanted to enjoy the mangoes alone so he decided to go down to the river to fight with that person and collect the mangoes from him.

Splash! Anansi fell down into the water. Holding his two mangoes firmly in his hands he started looking around. To his surprise there was no one else there. The swift currents carried Anansi away like a leaf. He struggled without success to get out of the river. Desperately, he released his hold on the mangoes and saw them floating away with the current.

Finally, exhausted and drenched, he came out of the river. His appetite for the mangoes had gone altogether! With bad grace he referred to them as 'sour mangoes'. With bitterness and anger Anansi went home, and that night he paid for his greed by having nothing to eat.

Being Greedy Chokes Anansi

Once upon a time, Kwaku Anansi lived in a country that had a queen who was also a witch. This queen had a secret name – the word 'five', and she didn't want anyone using it. It happened that she issued a decree that whoever used the word 'five' would fall down dead,

Now Anansi was a clever fellow and a hungry one too. Things had been especially bad because there was a famine in the land. Anansi decided to make a little house for himself by the side of the river, just near the point where everyone came to get water. He also made five yam hills next to his house. His plan was to call out to anyone who came along, 'I beg you to tell me how many yam hills I have here. I can't count very well.' He hoped that different animals would come up and say, 'One, two, three, four, five,' and then they would fall down dead. Then Anansi would take them and store them in his barrel and eat them, and that way he would always have lots of food, in hungry times and in times of plenty.

After some time, along came Guinea Fowl. Anansi said, 'I beg you, missus, tell me how many yam hills I have here.' So Guinea Fowl went and sat on one of the yam hills and said, 'One, two, three, four, and the one I'm sitting on!' Anansi said, 'Cho!' (sucking his teeth), 'you can't count right.' And Guinea Fowl moved to another hill and said, 'One, two, three, four, and the one I'm sitting on!' 'Cho! You don't count right at all' said Anansi.

'How do you count, then?' Guinea Fowl asked, a little confused by Anansi's strange behaviour. 'Why this way: one, two, three, four, FIVE!' And on saying this last word, Anansi fell down dead and Guinea Fowl ate him up.

Anansi and the Birds

Once upon a time, in the land where Kwaku Anansi lived, there was a big famine and all the animals were struggling to find enough to eat.

Meanwhile all the birds of the land were getting plenty to eat. Each day they would fly across the waters to a special island to feed on the cherry trees. The cherries were so big, sweet and juicy that when the birds ate them, the cherry juices would run down their beaks and stain all their feathers dark red.

Because it was an island, only the birds could easily get there. Every time Anansi heard the birds boasting about the juicy cherries, it made him want to go there more and more. But every time he asked to go, not one of the birds would offer to help. They would say: 'If God wanted you to go to Cherry Island, He would have made you a bird. Now go away and leave us alone.'

Anansi sat down and thought and thought until he came up with a plan. Finally he had an idea. When the birds returned from the island later that day, he asked every one of them for a feather. As this seemed such a small request, from Hummingbird to Weaver, every bird gave him one of their feathers.

The next morning, when the time came for the birds to return to Cherry Island, Anansi tied on the feathers. He then climbed up a tall cocon ut tree and jumped off and started to fly. Following all the birds, he flew until he reached the island. He landed in the largest cherry tree and he started to eat. And he ate and he ate and he ate!

Meanwhile the birds were murmuring about Anansi's greediness. They were worried that at the rate he was going there wouldn't be any cherries left for them. Anansi ignored their comments and continued eating. The more the birds murmured, the more angry they grew, until Weaver Bird said: 'Anansi, you are ungrateful. Look how we each lent you a feather to come here. Now you are eating all the cherries!'

Anansi just continued eating the cherries and ignoring the birds. So one by one the birds took back their feathers. Soon Anansi had none left. The birds flew back to the mainland at the end of the day and Anansi was left by himself on the island all night. The next day he had to swim the long, long, long way back home.

The Frangipani Maiden

This story is based on the Grimm's fairytale called 'Star Money' and is suitable for five- to eight-year-olds. Instead of the poor girl in the story, it uses a little bush spirit called the Frangipani Maiden. Taking an approach that seeks positive redress of greediness, it has a theme of giving and sharing. Note: the frangipani tree is most often found in tropical areas, and has a beautiful flower with waxy petals ranging in colour from white through pink and yellow to red.

It once happened that, in the bushland by the seashore, a little frangipani maiden was wandering all alone. The cold autumn winds had blown her far from her mother tree and she now had no home or family around her. The only clothes that she wore were the white and pink petals around her waist, the green leaves over her shoulders and the green leaves wrapped warmly on her head. The only food she had to eat were some wild raspberries that she had found along the sandy path.

But the little frangipani maiden was not worried or frightened. She knew that as long as she was thankful for the little she had, she would be taken care of and would always have enough.

As she wandered along the path, looking for a place to sit and eat her wild raspberries, she met a little bird who called out to her:

'I have no food, please give me something to eat'. Straight away the little frangipani maiden gave the bird her berries and went on her way.

Presently she saw a little mouse who called out to her:

'I have no hat, the wind is cold'. So the little frangipani maiden took off the green leaves that were warming her head, and gave her leaf hat to the mouse.

A little further on she met a spider who called out to her:

'I have no coat, the wind is cold'. The little frangipani maiden took off her leaf coat and gave it to the spider to make a little coat house.

Then she met a little ant, huddled by the pathway. The ant called out to her:

'I have no clothes, the wind is cold'. The little frangipani maiden took off her pink and white petals and built a little petal house for the ant to crawl inside.

Now the little frangipani maiden had nothing left. She had given away her food and all her clothes. But she was not worried or frightened. She knew that she would be taken care of. She continued on her way, and as it was starting to get dark, she soon found a place to sleep next to the sandy path amongst some leaves and grass.

While she slept, the stars in the heavens above danced and swirled. They swirled and danced, and danced and swirled, weaving for her a shining silken gown.

The little frangipani maiden woke to find herself wrapped in silver silk, with a golden shower falling all around her. At first she thought that the stars, which looked like pieces of glittering gold in the heavens, were falling down. But when the drops reached the ground, she saw they were real gold. She gathered them up and continued on her way. After this time, the little frangipani maiden never wanted for anything more for the rest of her life.

13

Irritating or Impatient

Pesky Pelican

Almost all parents have moments when their child is being annoying or irritating. It can happen at dinnertime when the child is hungry and the parent is tired. It can happen in the car on a long trip when the child is bored and the parent is stressed. At such moments a humorous poem can help relieve the situation.

A parent would be unlikely to know such a long poem by heart. I used to keep copies of selected poems on the fridge door to refer to when needed.

Sometimes just reading through the verses healed the problem, or at least changed the subject, and definitely offered a better approach than direct confrontation!

Pesky Pelican was a bird,
An annoying, irritating, pesky bird,
A bird that lived on the sandy shore,
A bird that always wanted more.
Even with all the fish in the sea,
Pesky Pelican wanted more for her tea!

Pesky Pelican could eat all day,
And always hunted in a pesky way,
She would poke around in holes and nests,
No animal or bird could ever rest,
No one was safe from her peskiness.

Her parents gave her warnings so sound,
Against her pesky poking around.
'You'll be sorry one day,
Mark what we say!
Go and catch fish in the waters blue,
This is what PEL-I-CANS should really do.'

But Pesky Pelican didn't care,
She just flapped her wings and flew up in the air.
She flapped her wings and made pesky sounds,
Then landed somewhere else on the ground.

Mother crabs could not leave their babies alone,
Could not safely leave their babes in their homes.
If they heard Pesky Pelican making her sounds.
They would cry out as PP came poking around:
'You'll be sorry one day,
Mark what we say!
Go and catch fish in the waters blue,
This is what PEL-I-CANS should really do.'

But Pesky Pelican didn't care,
She just flapped her wings and flew up in the air.
She flapped her wings and made pesky sounds,
Then landed somewhere else on the ground.

Mother birds could not leave their babies alone,
Could not safely leave their babes in their homes,
If they heard Pesky Pelican making her sounds.
They would cry out as PP came poking around:
'You'll be sorry one day,
Mark what we say!
Go and catch fish in the waters blue,
This is what PEL-I-CANS should really do.'

But Pesky Pelican didn't care,
She just flapped her wings and flew up in the air.
She flapped her wings and made pesky sounds,
Then landed somewhere else on the ground.

The fishermen could not leave their bags on the beach,
If they knew Pesky Pelican was close within reach,
If they heard Pesky Pelican making her sounds.
They would cry out as PP came poking around:
'You'll be sorry one day,
Mark what we say!
Go and catch fish in the waters blue,
This is what PEL-I-CANS should really do.'

But then, one day,
Mark what I say,
Pesky Pelican came unstuck,
Her behaviour had really run amuck,
In less time than a nod and a wink,
She carried her peskiness over the brink.

She was poking around near a fisherman's bag,
Having a Pesky Pelican look,
When she saw a fish that looked so fine,
Hanging in the air,
It looked so fine,
And she swallowed it whole,
With its hook and its line.

The hook and line were attached to a rod,
And the rod was attached to a fisherman's hand,
A fisherman standing close by on the sand.

Now Pesky Pelican had to care!
She couldn't flap her wings and fly up in the air,
She could only stand very still ... and despair!

But lucky the fisherman was a kind old man,
And good at helping pesky birds on the sand.
He gently pulled on the line with his hands ...
Slowly and gently he pulled with his hands,
Until up Pesky Pelican's throat slid the fish,
And landed plop in the fisherman's dish!

Pesky Pelican flapped her wings and flew high,
She flew up and across the bright blue sky,
She flapped her wings and flew high in the air,
Then out and over the ocean fair.
This time she didn't land back on the ground,
And she didn't make pesky pelican sounds.

Once she was alone and over the sea,
A different pelican she came to be.
She began to catch fish in the waters blue,
(Following her parents' good advice of course)
She did what PEL-I-CANS should really do!

Impatient Zebra

Originally written as a nature story for Kenyan children, this story is about an impatient zebra who has to learn to wait for his black stripes. It is based on the observation of baby zebras having golden brown stripes for their first year of life. Their stripes only turn black as they grow older. 'Impatient Zebra' is a therapeutic story for children and adults. For the adults it has a message of slowing down and allowing children time to be children.

Little Brown Zebra was not happy. He didn't want to have brown furry stripes like all the other baby zebras. He wanted to have black stripes like his mother and father and all his older brothers and sisters. He thought there was something wrong with him. Why were his stripes brown and white, when everybody in the whole world knew that zebras were supposed to be black and white?

Little Brown Zebra thought and thought about this all day long. In fact he couldn't think about anything else. His mother would get cross with him as he never seemed to be concentrating properly on what little zebras were supposed to be learning – important things like the best grasses to eat and how to sniff the air and tell if 'simba'[i] was close by. Instead he would mope around singing his impatient song:

> *I'm a little zebra and I'm feeling so down;*
> *My stripes should be black, but they are all brown.*

Little Brown Zebra was so concerned about his dilemma that he decided he was going to find a way to turn his brown stripes into black ones. He looked and looked around until he found some thick black mud by the edge of the dam. Then he tried to roll around in it, only letting the black mud get on his stripes. But you can imagine what happened – Little Brown Zebra ended up black all over, and looked more like a baby buffalo than a zebra. When his mother saw what he had done she sent him straight into the water to wash off the mud. After this his brown stripes seemed to be shining even more brightly.

So Little Brown Zebra continued to mope around for the rest of the day singing his impatient song:

> *I'm a little zebra and I'm feeling so down;*
> *My stripes should be black, but they are all brown.*

The next day he had a different idea. He found a burnt-out tree stump and started to rub the stripes on his back against the blackened wood. Stripe by stripe he kept on rubbing. This seemed to be working at first. Then Little Brown Zebra grew so excited that before he knew what he was doing he was rubbing too hard and he ended up with very sore patches all over his back. He had been rubbing his skin off altogether!

It took a long time for his skin to heal over, and all this time Little Brown Zebra continued to mope around singing his impatient song:

I'm a little zebra and I'm feeling so down;
My stripes should be black, but they are all brown.

His next idea was to try to stay under the shade of the acacia trees – at least this way his brown stripes looked darker than if he was out in the bright sunshine. But the grass didn't grow sweet and long in the shade of the trees, and Little Brown Zebra soon grew hungry.

After many hours of standing in the shade, he finally grew tired of being hungry. He was also growing tired of worrying about having brown stripes. It suddenly seemed more important to have a full tummy, so he left the shady trees and joined his family eating sweet grass on the sunny plains.

Some months later, he was travelling with his mother down to the river to have a cool drink. While he was standing on the riverbank, he looked down into the water, and to his surprise he saw that his stripes seemed to be the same colour as his mother's. He turned his head around to look at his stripy back, and sure enough, his stripy back had turned black! He wasn't a Little Brown Zebra anymore.

'What has happened to me?' he asked his mother. His mother smiled, nuzzled her nose into his neck, and whispered into his ear, 'You have grown. You are not a little zebra anymore.'

Little Zebra breathed a big sigh – of course, now he realised, all he had to do to turn his brown stripes into black ones was to GROW!

He galloped and gambolled round in circles singing a new song:

I'm a growing zebra and I'm happy to say,
my zebra stripes are black today!

i   'Simba' is the Kiswahili word for lion

14

Lazy

The Three Weaver Brothers

While living in the African bush I enjoyed watching the weaverbirds spending hours building their intricate nests. Their differing efforts reminded me of the timeless classic 'The Three Little Pigs' and so I re-wrote this story with an African theme. 'Kisulisuli' means 'a small whirlwind' (whirly-whirly) in Kiswahili.

Although it is not a story written to address a specific negative behaviour, it has general therapeutic use as it encourages concentrated work and commitment to a task. It was one of the most popular stories in the kindergarten in Nairobi the year it was written. Its positive effect was observed one day with one of the five-year-old boys who was prone to being quite lazy and not willing to finish tasks. He was overheard in creative playtime encouraging his friends to help him build a very strong house – just like the third weaver brother!

It was the first time I had observed this boy playing in a committed manner, and his concentrated work improved on a daily basis after this.

Once upon a time there were three weaver brothers who had grown old enough to fly from their parents' nest and build new homes.

'Goodbye,' said their mother, 'make sure your new home is high off the ground'.

'Goodbye,' said their father, 'make sure your new home is woven strong and sound'.

The first weaver brother landed on the low branch of an acacia tree. 'This will do me,' he said, not bothering to look further. He then started to collect some twigs and grass to weave his home.

It was hardly finished when along came a tall giraffe and with a single lick of his long tongue he swallowed the branch and nest, all in one. The first weaver brother just managed to fly off in time.

The second weaver brother flew around for a while, then landed on the high branch of another acacia tree. 'This will do me,' he said, and started to collect some twigs and grass to weave his home. After a short while he grew tired of his work and began to quickly fix his twigs and grass together. He didn't bother to make it strong and sound.

It was hardly finished when along came a Kisulisuli Wind and blew around the acacia tree. 'I'll whirl and I'll twirl and I'll swirl your house down' said the Kisulisuli. But the second weaver brother just laughed and said 'Go ahead little Kisulisuli, you don't scare me.'

So the Kisulisuli whirled and the Kisulisuli twirled, and sure enough it swirled the nest right out of the tree and down to the ground. The second weaver brother just managed to fly off in time.

The third weaver brother landed in another acacia tree. Before he started to weave his nest, he remembered the advice his mother had given him and looked for the highest branch of all. Finally he found a branch right in the middle at the top of the tree, far too high for the giraffe's tongue to reach. This will do me, he said, and started to collect some twigs and grass to weave his home.

This weaver brother was a hard worker – he had listened to the advice of his father. He took a very long time to find the right twigs and grass, and he took a very long time to weave them together – in and out, over and under, in and out – all the time singing as he worked:

Here I am, a busy little weaver, busy little weaver, busy little weaver,
Here I am, a busy little weaver, weaving my nest all day.

Finally after many, many days of hard work, his new home was high off the ground and was woven strong and sound. When it was ready, along came a Kisulisuli Wind and blew around the acacia tree. 'I'll whirl and I'll twirl and I'll swirl your house down' said the Kisulisuli, but the third weaver brother just laughed and said 'Go ahead little Kisulisuli, you don't scare me.'

So the Kisulisuli whirled and twirled, and it twirled and it whirled. But no matter how hard it tried, it wasn't able to swirl the strong nest out of the tree. Eventually the Kisulisuli whirled away to find something else to annoy or destroy.

The third weaver brother lined his strong nest with some feathers to make a soft bed, then he crawled inside and had a long rest. When he awoke, he found his two brothers waiting outside his nest. Seeing the wonderful home their brother had made, they had come to ask if he had room for them too.

The third weaver brother told them that he needed space for a wife and new babies to live. He sent his other two brothers off to try once again to make their own homes, saying to them: 'Make sure your new home is high off the ground. Make sure your new home is woven strong and sound.'

This time the other brothers listened to this good advice. Soon the bushland was ringing with their weaving songs as they busily made nests high off the ground and wove them strong and sound:

> *Here we are, the busy little weavers,*
> *busy little weavers, busy little weavers,*
> *Here we are, the busy little weavers, weaving nests all day.*

The Fisherman

A 'Lou' tale from the shores of Lake Victoria (Western Kenya), suitable for ages 6 – 8. This consequential story deals with the theme of 'laziness', and is included by permission of the author, Elizabeth Aoko.

Once upon a time there was an old fisherman who lived by himself in a little hut on the lakeshore. Every day, early in the morning, before the sunrise, the old man walked down to the edge of the water. There he put his little canoe into the waves, climbed in, and with a long rod he pushed the canoe out into the deep waters of the lake. Then he cast his fishing net, and, leaving it in the water, he sailed back to the shore to wait. Sitting in the shade of the tree, he would fill in his time by singing:

Nyamgodho wnod Omaber; Nejachani, ncayudo dhako majakibaya.
(Nyamgodho son of Omaber, he was poor but he met a fairy lady)

Then, after a while, the old man would get back into his canoe, and sail through the waves into the deep water to pull up his net.

One day, when he was pulling in his net, he was surprised to find that it was unusually heavy. 'This is a big catch of fish' he thought to himself as he pulled and pulled on the ropes. Eventually he was able to pull the net beside his boat. To his surprise he found that it was not full of fish, but inside was a beautiful young lady.

'Don't shake me out of your net,' she pleaded with the fisherman. 'Please carry me home with you'. The fisherman happily agreed, and the beautiful lady climbed aboard the canoe and sailed with the fisherman to the shore. Once they were ashore, the old man lit a fire, cooked some sweet potatoes and made some tea.

After they had shared a meal together, the young lady asked the man to build a boma (fenced yard) for some cows, goats, sheep and chickens. For three days the old fisherman worked hard, sawing and tying and hammering, sawing and tying and hammering, sawing and tying and hammering – building a strong home for animals to live in.

When the boma was ready, the young lady walked back to the lakeshore, and called out across the water:

Dhoga biabia; dhoga biabia
(All my animals come out of the sea)

Suddenly many cows came out of the waves and walked up onto the shore and followed her into the boma.

The next day the young lady walked back to the lakeshore and called out again:

Dhoga biabia; dhoga biabia

This time many goats came out of the waves and walked up onto the shore and followed her into the boma.

The next day the young lady walked back to the lakeshore and called out again:

Dhoga biabia; dhoga biabia

This time many sheep came out of the waves and walked up onto the shore and followed her into the boma.

The next day the young lady walked back to the lakeshore and called out again:

Dhoga biabia; dhoga biabia

This time many chickens came out of the waves and walked up onto the shore and followed her into the boma.

The old fisherman was so happy. He had a beautiful lady to share his house and many animals in his boma. But, as time went by, the man started to get lazy and lie around. He stopped attending to the jobs that were needed to look after the house and the animals. At first he forgot to feed the cows, then the goats, then the sheep and then the chickens. And then, when the boma fence needed repairs, he didn't want to bother with this.

The young lady was not pleased that the man was growing lazy and not taking care of her animals. So she sat down one day under the mango tree to think about what could be done. Finally she decided it was time for her to return to the waters of the lake where she had lived before.

Early the next morning, after the sun had risen, she stood at the boma gate and once again sang her song to her animals:

Dhoga biabia; dhoga biabia; Dhoga biabia; dhoga biabia;
Dhoga biabia; dhoga biabia.

One by one all the cows, the goats, the sheep and the chickens started to walk out through the gate and down to the water. The old fisherman tried to chase and grab hold of the animals, but his lazy legs could not move fast enough to catch them. Slowly he followed them to the lakeshore, just in time to watch the young lady disappear into the waves followed by all the cows, goats, sheep and chickens. He stood at the edge of the water, watching helplessly as he listened to the lady's song slowly fade away:

Dhoga biabia; dhoga biabia [sing very softly]

Sadly he turned and walked back home, and was surprised to find that the boma that he had built for the animals had also disappeared. All that was left was his little hut, just like before.

From that time on, the old fisherman continued to fish in the lake. Every day, early in the morning, before the sunrise, he walked down to the edge of the water. There he put his little canoe into the waves, climbed in, and with a long rod he pushed the canoe out into the deep waters of the lake. Then he cast his fishing net, and, leaving it in the water, he sailed back to the shore to wait.

Sitting in the shade of the tree, he would fill in his time by singing:

Nyamgodho wnod Omaber; Nejachani, ncayudo dhako majakibaya.
Then, after a while, the old man would get back into his canoe, and
sail through the waves into the deep water to pull up his net and
collect his catch of fish. He never saw the young lady again. But
sometimes, on days when the wind was still and all was quiet, he was
sure he could hear a faint song coming up from the deep:

Dhoga biabia, dhoga biabia; Dhoga biabia, dhoga biabia

15

Noisy or Disruptive

Noisy Gnome Story

*This story has the potential to be used with many different age groups.
It was written during a year when my five-year-old group was extremely
rowdy in their play. I had observed some of the shyer children having difficulty coping with the noise levels, and my assistant and I were also struggling with the daily noise. The light-hearted humour of the story gave us
a way of addressing the challenge. In fact one of my quiet little boys, who
hardly spoke in the bigger group, was heard calling out to the noisy boys
in their dens: 'Dear oh dear, I can't bear it any more, my rub-a-dub ears
are much too sore!'*

*The little rhyme was used by the teachers for many weeks after the
story to suggest quieter play. It was a successful approach, and certainly more productive than simply saying 'Play more quietly please.' The
emphasis on 'noise' in the story also helped bring an awareness of the
pleasures of 'quiet' to the room. I extended the story by bringing in many
river stones to clean and polish. The children grew to love quiet moments when they could listen to the stones 'singing'.*

Once upon a time there were four little gnomes and they lived together in their rocky cave home. Three of the gnome brothers were like peas in a pod – they looked alike, they dressed alike, and most of all they loved to make lots of noise. With their picks and hammers they would work together all day long, digging for crystals and making a very noisy song.

There was Hump-dunk and he went hump, dunk, hump, dunk.

There was Brink-a-brac and he went brink-brink brac, brink-brink brac.

There was Clinken-clank and he went clinkety-clank, clinkety-clank.

Together they sounded like this:

Hump, dunk, brink-brink brac, clinkety-clank; Hump, dunk, brink-brink brac, clinkety-clank; Hump, dunk, brink-brink brac, clinkety-clank.

There was a fourth gnome brother and he was very different from all the others. He looked different, he dressed differently, and his work was very different. His name was Rub-a-dub-gnome and his job was to polish the crystal stones that had been dug out of the rock cave by his brothers.

Rub-a-dub-gnome didn't like noise! He would sit in the corner of the cave with his polishing rag and work away quietly. He rubbed and polished the crystal stones until they shone with silver light. Whenever it happened that his brothers were away for a while and all was quiet in the cave, Rub-a-dub-gnome was sure that he could hear the stones singing.

The four gnome brothers lived together and worked together in their rocky cave home. But it was a very difficult life for Rub-a-dub-gnome. He was always calling out to his noisy brothers, 'Please, please, not so much noise, my Rub-a-dub ears are getting sore.'

But Hump-dunk, Brink-a-brac and Clinken-clank loved making noise. They just kept on digging and hammering and making a hump, dunk, brink-brink brac, clinkety-clank sound, all day long!

One day Hump-dunk, Brink-a-brac and Clinken-clank were making such a racket that Rub-a-dub-gnome had to stop work and sit and hold his hands over his ears. So no more stones were polished for the rest of the day.

The next day, as the hump, dunk, brink-brink brac, clinkety-clank sound continued just as loud as before, Rub-a-dub-gnome decided he had had enough.

'Dear oh dear' he exclaimed, 'I can't bear it any more.

My Rub-a-dub ears are much too sore!'

Rub-a-dub-gnome gathered up his polishing rags and all his stones and put them into a large sack. He said goodbye to his noisy brothers and left his cave home in the hill. With his sack on his back he set out to look for another home where it would be quiet and still.

From that day to this, Rub-a-dub-gnome has lived by himself. But often his brothers come to visit him in his quiet cave and bring him new stones to polish, and sometimes he goes to visit his brothers in their noisy cave home.

When the three brothers come to visit Rub-a-dub-gnome they try very hard to be quiet, and when Rub-a-dub-gnome visits his brothers he tries very hard to enjoy their noise. But he never stays for very long!

Never-Get-Enough By Sandra Frain (B.C.S, M.S.C)

This story was written 'on the spot' by a Canadian early years teacher when a 5-year-old boy labelled 'mildly autistic' was creating havoc in pre-school. He was threatening other children and the teachers, and was basically in control of the mood in the room. Sandra's colleague said, 'I think he needs a story about an animal.'

They immediately set up benches in a diamond shape in the middle of the room. Sandra wanted a 'different' set-up from the usual storytelling place as this was not the usual story time. She swooped the boy up in her arms and cradled him and they called the others to sit down for a surprise. Sandra began after a quick silent prayer and a deep breath. She recounts having no idea what she was embarking on – she just let the story tell itself. ... The children were completely quiet and engrossed in the story. The boy was subdued too. According to both teachers it seemed a transformative experience.

Since this time, Sandra has used the same story for a boy who bit another child, and for when she feels a particular child, or the whole group, needs to be 'brought in' to themselves. The story gives a sense of warm enclosure and protection.

Once upon a time there was a puppy that lived with his brothers and sisters and his mummy in a kennel. Never-Get-Enough was the last to be born in the litter. He was the runt of the litter.

Never-Get-Enough whimpered and whined when he got squashed under his big fluffy roly-poly brothers and sisters. They were always rolling around, biting each other's necks, and tumbling over each other.

Whenever their mummy lay down with them his brothers and sisters would clamour over each other to get a teat to suckle milk from. Never-Get-Enough had to wait until one of his brothers or sisters had fallen asleep and he could nuzzle in. He would suck and suck but he couldn't get enough sweet warm milk before Mummy got up for a stretch. Then he would be dropped from her belly – cold and hungry.

One day a lady came to visit the kennel. 'I'm looking for a nice little puppy' she said. Never-Get-Enough looked up at the lady looming over the wall of the kennel. His brothers and sister were busy rolling and clamouring and yipping and yapping.

The silver-haired lady looked right into Never-Get-Enough's eyes and she scooped him up in her hands and put him right next to her heart.

'I would like this puppy' she said. The silver haired lady put Never-Get-Enough into the cosy red pocket that was over her heart. She put her soft warm hand over his head.

'I like his puppy smell,' she said as she breathed him in. She put her finger to his mouth. Never-Get-Enough closed his eyes and put his sharp little teeth and his wet tongue around her finger.

'I will look after him,' she said to his mummy. Never-Get-Enough snuggled into the pocket and fell fast asleep as the lady walked home and he rocked back and forth and back and forth in her cosy heart-pocket.

Garden of Birds

This story was written for a university student who was enrolled in my Storytelling unit but proved to be too 'talkative' on our internet 'chat' line. One of the other students commented on this person's dominance of the chat space, and the talkative student then emailed me privately for some help with learning to listen.

The story could easily be used with children aged five and older who are too talkative in class.

Once upon a time there was a bird that sang so beautifully she filled the garden with her birdsong from morning to night.

Many other birds lived in this garden but they weren't able to sing over the top of the beautiful songbird. Even if they tried to sing, their sounds just seemed to disappear into nowhere. The songbird filled the air and the garden with her non-stop singing and there was no room for any other songs. If the other birds wanted to practise their singing, they had to fly out of the garden and high up into the mountains where there was no competition.

One day, however, the beautiful songbird grew very sick and was unable to sing any more. She rested in her nest, day after day. The garden around her was very quiet, and each day when the birds returned from the mountains they wondered what had happened.

One by one the other birds began to stay behind in the garden and take turns to sing. Soon the garden was filled with the sound of many birds with many different songs.

The sick bird was very surprised to listen to so many other birds – all their songs were very different and very beautiful. She had never heard anything like this before. The more she lay in her nest and listened to the new sounds the stronger she grew. The singing was helping to heal her.

Soon the songbird was feeling better and she was able to sing once more. But she decided to sing only every so often and not all the time so that she could enjoy the songs of the other birds. She was also learning so many new bird sounds by listening to the others, and gradually her own singing became richer and better because of this.

As time passed this garden became well-known for its beautiful bird songs and its rich variety of bird sounds. People came from far and wide to spend time here to walk, sit and listen. Some even found healing in such a wonderful place.

16

Pinching, Hurting or Fighting

Cranky Crab

A child therapist used this story with a four-year-old girl who often pinched other children. Gloves of the child's favourite colour became a strengthening 'prop'. After hearing the story, the child wanted to wear the gloves and keep her pinching fingers warm and cosy inside. The story helped the child get the message in an imaginative and fun way, and the problem was slowly healed.

Parents, therapists and teachers could use this story theme for other kinds of aggressive behaviour, using a different animal in place of the crab (e.g. a scratching cat).

Little Crab was not very popular with the beach-boy group.

His friends were tired of him always being in a cranky mood and using his claws to nip and hurt them.

One day, Turtle decided to call a meeting to put a stop to it all.

Octopus, Starfish, and Seagull came along to give their ideas.

'We should cut his claws right off', said Octopus, who was still nursing one of his tentacles from a nasty nip last week.

'Perhaps we should glue them together,' suggested Starfish, who now had two shorter star legs because of Crab's bad behaviour.

'Or tie them behind Crab's back – with a very strong piece of string!' cried Seagull, whose foot had been bitten by Crab just that morning.

'But what if we can help Crab learn to stop hurting us', said Turtle, who always tried to be the most understanding of all the beach friends.

'That's a very nice idea, Turtle, but what do we do while he is learning?' all the friends cried out together. They had had enough of

Crab's cranky moods. They also didn't believe that Crab would ever be able to change his hurting ways.

Turtle wandered slowly backwards and forwards along the sand, thinking in his wise turtle way. Suddenly he stopped next to a pile of seaweed. 'I have an idea' he announced to the group. 'I will knit some thick seaweed mittens for Crab to wear on his claws. These might help him learn to be more careful.'

Turtle was very excited by his idea. He went straight back to his cave in the rock pool to get his pair of driftwood knitting needles. Meanwhile the other beach friends reluctantly agreed to collect some long strands of seaweed. When Turtle returned, there was a big pile of seaweed ready for him, and he set to work knitting a pair of mittens for Crab to wear on his claws.

Just as he finished the second mitten, Crab arrived. 'What's happening, guys?' asked Crab. Of course he was very curious to know what his friends had been up to all morning!

Quickly Turtle said, 'We have a present for you Crab'. And he held out the mittens for Crab to try them on. Well, Crab was so surprised, you could have knocked him over with a fish-eagle feather. Never before had anyone given him a gift. Straight away he pulled the mittens on over his claws, and they fitted perfectly!

For the rest of the day the beach friends played together – with no nipping and no hurting, just happily together. Crab's friends could not believe it. And Crab could not believe it. You see, for Crab something else happened that day. Once his claws were both tucked away inside the mittens, held together in a warm and cosy kind of way, he didn't feel as cranky as he used to feel.

Of course, when Crab was hungry he had to take his mittens off so he could hunt in the rock pools for his dinner. But before playing with his friends again, he would always put the mittens back over his sharp claws. The mittens seemed to help him feel happy, and they certainly helped him be more careful.

However, seaweed mittens cannot last forever. One day the mittens were so full of holes that they simply fell off Crab's claws and the waves washed them out to sea. Fortunately, by this time, Crab had learnt to use his claws only for hunting and eating. He now knew how to keep them tightly closed when he was playing with his friends.

The beach friends were very impressed by how wise Turtle had been. From that day on, whenever they had a problem to sort out, they would always ask for his suggestion. And more often than not, Turtle's idea was the best one.

The Enormous Nail

A traditional Xhosa story researched by Maria Msebenzi and re-written by the author. It is suitable for age seven and over.

Once upon a time there was a young boy called Maxabela. This boy had an unusually long fingernail, and nobody could get him to cut it off.

Maxabela wanted to keep his very large and very long nail. He enjoyed using it to pinch and scratch other children. His nail was like a weapon!

His parents were both annoyed and concerned about their son's behaviour. But when they asked him to stop hurting other children, Maxabela would not listen to them.

The days and weeks went by and Maxabela kept on with his hurting behaviour. Finally his parents decided that something needed to be done. Together they made a plan.

In a field far away from their village, they built a little thatched house for Maxabela. When it was ready, they told him that he must stay there to watch over the crops and vegetables. Maxabela was very excited about this, as he knew that his enormous nail was going to work for him and make sure he had enough to eat.

As soon as his parents left him alone, Maxabela set off to the garden and used his long strong nail to help him dig up some vegetables. He took them back to his little house and put them to cook in a pot on the fire. Soon the delicious smell of the cooked food attracted a passing giant.

Maxabela heard a big gruff voice outside his door. 'Hey Maxabela, whose food is this?'

'It is mine' called back Maxabela, trembling with fear.

'Don't you mean, it is mine?' cried the giant, and he pushed open the door, came inside and ate up all the food. Then he went on his way.

That night Maxabela went to bed with an empty stomach.

The next morning Maxabela set off to the garden again and used his nail to help dig up some more vegetables. He took them back to his little house and put them to cook in a pot on the fire. Soon the delicious smell of the cooked food attracted the giant.

Maxabela heard a big gruff voice outside his door. 'Hey Maxabela, whose food is this?'

'It is mine' called back Maxabela.

'Don't you mean, it is mine?' cried the giant, and he pushed open the door and came inside.

This time Maxabela decided he didn't want the giant to eat his food, and he started to fight back. He tried to use his enormous nail to pinch the giant, but the giant's skin was as hard as stone and caused Maxabela's nail to break off at his fingertip. The giant ate up all the food, then left Maxabela's house with the broken nail in his hand.

That night, under cover of darkness, the giant delivered the broken nail to Maxabela's parents' home. The next morning the mother found her son's nail on her doorstep. She quickly walked across the fields to visit her son and found him trembling inside his little thatched house.

Maxabela's mother hugged her son and took him back home with her. Since this time Maxabela has never hurt anybody again, and he plays happily with his friends.

Jeremy and the Magic Sticks

This story was written to introduce a series of knitting lessons to a class of aggressive and unsettled eight-year-olds. See Chapter Three for an explanation of the use and effect of this story.

Jeremy was not a happy boy. Nothing could please him and nobody could make him smile. He almost seemed to enjoy being grumpy and hurtful. His mother and his teacher would shake their heads in despair – they didn't know how to handle him and how to help him co-operate.

Today Jeremy was particularly grumpy. It was holiday time and he was at home on the farm all by himself. His sisters were away at the coast with friends, so he had nobody to tease and nothing to do. His mother was busy harvesting on the vegetable patch. She had no time to pay attention to his 'down-in-the-dumps' grumps.

Round and round the house Jeremy walked, hitting walls and banging cupboard doors, then out on to the veranda to find the dog and pull his tail. In the garden he threw gum nuts at the chickens then, armed with a handful of pebbles from the driveway, he headed off in the direction of the stream at the bottom of the farm.

From a high position on a large rock, Jeremy busied himself trying to hit every tree and flower that grew by the water. He then spied a little grass house amongst the fern bracken. 'My silly sisters probably built this', he thought to himself, laughing about their crazy idea of making houses for the fairies to live in. Picking up an extra large pebble he hurled it at the little house.

To his absolute amazement, as soon as the pebble hit the grassy roof, out jumped a tiny man, about the size of Jeremy's hand. Jeremy almost fell off his rock in surprise. He was even more surprised to see the little man coming through the grass towards him. And the little man didn't look very happy. In fact he looked extremely upset! For a moment, Jeremy actually felt a little frightened.

The little man came right up to the rock, and with his hands on his hips and a very cross voice he said, 'Who dares to throw giant rocks on my house?'

Jeremy opened his mouth to argue that it was not him, but instead he found himself saying, 'I'm very sorry, but it was me.'

With this apology, the little man calmed down somewhat, and asked Jeremy why he didn't have anything better to do with his time. 'Are you perhaps bored?' he asked the bewildered boy.

Now this was a new experience for Jeremy. He was so used to everyone getting cross with him, and not ever asking him questions. In fact Jeremy had never even heard of the word 'bored' before. In an unusually polite manner, he answered, 'Excuse me, little man, what do you mean by the word 'bored'?'

The little man hopped up onto the rock and sat down next to Jeremy. 'Being bored' he said, 'means not knowing how to be busy … and not knowing how to be busy is a terrible, terrible thing! Indeed, if I didn't keep my hands busy making things and fixing things my fingers would probably grow cold and just fall right off!'

On saying this, the little man reached out, right in front of Jeremy's eyes, and took hold of a shaft of golden sunlight shining down through the branches next to the rock. With very quick fingers he started to knot it and loop it and make it into a long golden chain. 'Look at this' he said, 'during the day I keep myself busy collecting extra sunlight from the hot summer days. Watch how I can knot it into a long golden chain to store away for cold winter nights.'

Jeremy watched with fascination as the little man's fingers worked quickly with the golden thread of light. When the chain was finished, the little man popped it into his pocket. Then he looked up at Jeremy and said, 'Young man, this is exactly what you need to do. If your fingers were working like mine, doing busy finger work, then they wouldn't have time to throw stones, would they? Show me what your fingers can do.'

Jeremy showed a few funny finger movements that made the little elf man laugh out loud. He reached out to take hold of another shaft of golden light and handed it to Jeremy. 'Show me how you can tie a knot' he said.

Jeremy proudly tied a little knot in the golden thread. 'Well done! Now tie a knot onto this branch, and I will teach you how to make long chains with your thread.'

The lesson continued for some time. Finally the little man suggested Jeremy return home to practise with threads from his mother's wool basket.

'Come back to this rock tomorrow and I will teach you how to work with magic sticks to make many more things'. On saying this, the little man disappeared into the tall grasses, leaving Jeremy to ponder the exciting events of the morning.

When Jeremy reached home he asked his mother for some scraps of wool. Needless to say, his mother was very impressed with the sudden change of behaviour in her son. She was especially delighted to watch him busy that night making long wool chains. She took out her sewing basket and helped him sew the chains onto a round piece of felt. Jeremy proudly put his new spiral mat on the table next to his bed, and that night both Jeremy and his mother slept very well.

The next day Jeremy returned to the rock for a second lesson with the little man. This time, before his lesson began, he was sent to look for two smooth sticks. When he returned with his sticks, the little man helped him sharpen two ends on the rough rock and find two gum nuts for the other ends. Then from his pocket he pulled out his own pair of magic sticks and set about showing the most amazing work with a long golden thread.

The work was called 'knitting' and as the little man knitted he sang a little song:

In, over, out and off we sail, to weave a magic golden veil.

Jeremy couldn't wait to start using his magic sticks. He needed several lessons before he could knit as beautifully as the little man but every day he practised and practised with his mother's wool. Soon his knitting had grown long enough to take it off the needles and sew into a little hat.

By the time his sisters returned from their holiday, Jeremy had knitted two hats for their dolls and a scarf for his mother. Of course his sisters wanted to learn how to make things with magic sticks, and Jeremy proudly offered to be their knitting teacher. He never saw the little man again, but the little man had taught him something he would never forget for the rest of his life – how to keep his hands busy making beautiful things.

Jeremy's mother and teacher never knew about the little man, but they were sure an angel must have paid the farm a visit that year!

The Beautiful Queen

Sometimes children's aggressive behaviour is directly connected with their stressed, depressed or anxious parent and/or teacher. I wrote the following story for a single mother of three angry, fighting children. The mother had no feeling of self-worth and needed help to rediscover her beauty. Not only did the story help the mother feel good about herself, but after reading it many times she decided to read it to her children (aged 13, 9 and 5). They all wanted to hear it again and again. Harmony re-entered the house during the newly established story ritual.

There was once a queen who lived in a castle with many children. This queen was wise and ruled her kingdom very well. This queen was also very beautiful. When her children were young they loved to sit on soft cushions around her throne, listen to her beautiful singing and look up at her beautiful face.

However, as the children grew older, they started to fight and argue and there was much yelling and shouting in the castle – so much so that the queen, whose ears only liked to hear beautiful sounds, started to wrap herself up in many coloured veils, around her head, and around her shoulders, all the while trying to cover her ears, trying to keep out the loud noises. The queen did not like harsh and loud noise, and as the fighting and shouting grew louder she would add more and more veils to protect her ears from the ugly sounds. She didn't know what else to do! The fighting and arguing continued and the children grew used to seeing their mother all wrapped up in coloured veils, with only her sad but beautiful eyes looking out at them. After many years it happened that the children forgot what their mother really looked like.

As the fighting and arguing grew worse, the queen also found a way to escape the children and their unbearable noises. Sometimes she would creep out of the castle and go down to the deep stream at the bottom of the garden. Here she would cross the water over the many stepping stones and then wander in the forest. She knew the children could not follow her into the forest as the stepping stones were magic ones. They only appeared when they heard her sing to them, and then disappeared again after she had crossed over.

Oh how this queen loved the forest! She would wander for hours along the paths beneath the shady trees, enjoying the peaceful forest sounds, collecting wild flowers and watching the animals and birds. Her favourite place was a deep green pool at the bottom of a sparkling waterfall. The pool was surrounded by rock gardens. Here many pink and white orchids grew in the golden sunlight that filtered down through the surrounding tall trees. The queen would sit on the rocks, and weave flower chains. On hot sunny days she would take off all her veils and swim in the cool green water.

One day when the queen was walking in the forest the children were out playing in the garden with their golden ball. One of the children kicked the ball so high that it landed at the bottom of the garden and rolled into the deep water. The fast flowing stream took the golden ball and it disappeared round the corner and into the forest. The children started to fight and argue about this, but no matter how much they argued and shouted, they realised that the golden ball would not come back unless someone fetched it.

As the golden ball was the favourite of all their toys, the older children who could swim decided that they would follow the ball down the stream and fetch it back. So they dived into the water and before long they were swimming under tall, shady trees, and in and around rocks and low hanging branches. The golden ball kept bobbing along ahead of them, all the way through the forest, until it reached a waterfall that fell far below into a deep green pool. The children stopped on a rock just before the waterfall and carefully reached out and looked over the edge. What they saw took their breath away. Sitting on the rocks far down below, amongst pink and white orchid flowers, was the most beautiful lady they had ever seen. This beautiful lady was playing with their golden ball, throwing it into the air and catching it again. As the children watched, she threw the golden ball into the water, dived in after it and continued to play and swim.

For a long time the children sat on the rocks at the top of the waterfall, not making a noise in case the lady should hear them and be frightened away. They watched till she had finished swimming and started to dress herself. To their amazement, they saw her wrap many veils around her, just like their mother the queen would wear. 'Perhaps she is a queen – perhaps veils are the clothes that all queens wear', they wondered as they watched her getting dressed. Then they saw her pick up the golden ball and follow a pathway that led away from the pool and deep into the forest. Before long she had disappeared from sight.

The children decided it was time to get home. Fortunately they found a path that followed the stream back through the forest to their side of the garden, a path they had never noticed before. On the way back nobody said a word. They were all busy with their own thoughts about the beautiful lady – who could she be, they wondered? Perhaps she was the queen of the forest? And if so, where did she live? They all knew that they wanted to see her again, she was so beautiful.

When they returned they told their brothers and sisters about what they had seen, and of course the younger children also wanted to see the beautiful forest lady. The next day all the children crept along the newly found path that led all the way through the forest to the top of the waterfall. There they waited, quietly lying on top of the rocks and peering over the edge so that they could see the green pool below. Before long the beautiful lady arrived, still carrying their golden ball. She took off all her veils and sat on the rocks, smelling the orchid flowers. Then she dived into the water and started to swim and play with the ball. For a long time all the children sat together on the waterfall watching the beautiful lady (whom they now thought must really be the forest queen), and then they crept back up the path and all the way home.

For many weeks the children went every day to the waterfall, and the more they journeyed into the forest the less fighting and arguing there was back at the castle. The children not only enjoyed watching the beautiful forest queen, but also the quiet of the forest and all the wonderful forest sounds.

Then one day, when they arrived at the waterfall, they waited and waited for the forest queen to appear at the pool below, but the whole day went by and nobody came. As it was getting dark they decided it was time to return, and sadly they followed the path towards home and arrived back at the castle just in time for dinner. The queen was sitting on her throne at the end of the large dining table where they all shared their meals – they were worried that she would ask them where they had been, but she said nothing. The children all sat down and ate their dinner and as nobody knew what to talk about nobody said anything. So the meal was shared in silence.

After they had finished eating, the queen surprised them all by asking if she could play ball with them. The children were busy trying to think of an excuse for why they didn't have a ball to play with. Then, from under the folds of her gown, the queen lifted out a beautiful golden ball, just like their beautiful golden ball. She then slowly started to take off her coloured veils, until her face was in full view. Now the children saw that the forest queen and their mother were one and the same person! They came close and sat on the soft cushions on the floor around her throne. Then the queen started to sing, just as beautifully as they remembered from long ago when they were little children. As she sang she threw the golden ball to each one of them in turn:

Up in the sky my ball so high,
Landing like a butterfly,
Gold as the sun, light as the air,
Come back to me – my ball so fair.

A Bag of Nails

This consequential story arrived in my email inbox via a story-chat line, an anonymous gem. It has a very powerful message for anger and aggression for primary school classes and beyond into adulthood, and could be used as the basis for a class or family discussion.

Once upon a time there was a little boy with a bad temper. His father gave him a bag of nails and told him that every time he lost his temper, he should hammer a nail in the fence. The first day the boy had driven 39 nails into the fence. But gradually, the number of nails per day dwindled. He discovered it was easier to keep his temper than drive those nails into the fence.

Finally the day came when the boy didn't lose his temper at all. He proudly told his father about it and the father suggested that the boy now pull out one nail for each day that he was able to keep his temper.

The days passed and the young boy was finally able to tell his father that all the nails were gone. The father took his son by the hand and led him to the fence.

'You have done well, my son, but look at the holes in the fence. The fence will never be the same. When you say things in anger, they leave a scar just like this one. If you put a knife in a man and draw it out, it won't matter how many times you say "I'm sorry", the wound is still there.'

17

Shy or Introverted

A Little Boy Went Sailing

Suitable for ages three to five, this story was written to encourage shy and/ or 'clinging' children to explore their pre-school or home garden – it can be modified depending on the adventures possible in the garden, whether at school or at home.

There was once a little boy (just about your size!) who wanted to have some adventures, so he climbed into his sailing boat and set sail across the sparkling blue sea. He hadn't sailed very far when he reached an island covered with giant rocks. He left his boat on the shore and started to climb the rocks – he climbed up and down, and up and down, and all around – but after a while he grew tired of playing on the rocks:

'Climbing giant rocks is lots of fun, but I want more adventures under the sun' he said, and climbed back into his boat and kept sailing over the sparkling blue sea.

Soon he came to an island covered with golden sand. Luckily he had his red spade with him, so he left his boat on the shore and started to play in the sand – he dug holes and rivers and tunnels, he made roads, and he built castles – but after a while he grew tired of digging in the sand:

'Digging in the sand is lots of fun, climbing giant rocks is lots of fun, but I want more adventures under the sun' he said, and climbed back into his boat and kept sailing over the sparkling blue sea.

Soon he came to an island covered with tall green banana trees. On one tree was a bunch of ripe yellow bananas. As he was feeling quite hungry this was just what the little boy needed. Leaving his boat by the shore, he walked to the tree and picked two bananas and sat down in the shade of the tree and ate them both. Then he said:

'Eating bananas is lots of fun, digging in the sand is lots of fun, climbing giant rocks is lots of fun, but I want more adventures under the sun' and climbed back into his boat and kept sailing over the sparkling blue sea.

Soon he came to an island where there was a deep green pool. He left his boat by the shore and paddled in the cool waters (he was feeling very hot by now!) For a long time he paddled and splashed in the water, but after a while he grew tired of playing in the water:

'Splashing in cool water is lots of fun, eating bananas is lots of fun, digging in the sand is lots of fun, climbing giant rocks is lots of fun, but I want more adventures under the sun' he said, and he climbed back into his boat and kept sailing over the sparkling blue sea.

Soon he came to an island that was covered with forest. Leaving his boat on the shore he followed a little path through the shady trees until he came to a clearing. In the middle of the clearing, built of logs and branches, was a beautiful bush castle – it had a little cubby house and lots of ladders, and a slippery dip to slide down and a swing to swing on. So the little boy started to play on the bush castle – he played in the cubby, he climbed the ladders, he 'whooshed' down the slide, he swung high and low. But after a while he said:

'Playing on the bush castle is lots of fun, splashing in cool water is lots of fun, eating bananas is lots of fun, digging in the sand is lots of fun, climbing giant rocks is lots of fun, but now I am so tired (YAWN), I don't want any more adventures under the sun. And when I am tired and need to rest, my little bed-boat is what I like best.'

So he climbed back into his boat and sailed all the way home. His mother was waiting for him. She gently lifted him into his little bed and tucked a soft blue blanket around him. Then she sang him a lullaby – it went like this:

> *A little boy went sailing across the sparkling sea*
> *He had so many things to do, so many things to see.*
> *And when the day was over, he sailed his way back home*
> *And snug inside his bed-boat, through dreamland he did roam.*

By the time his mother had finished singing, the little boy was fast, fast asleep.

Strawberry Shy and Raspberry Wild

This story was written to encourage a self-conscious eight-year-old to stop hiding under her clothes at the beach, put on her swimmers and come out into the sun to swim and play. Although the story didn't have any noticeable effect on the child (apart from her liking the story very much) there was positive feedback from her parents. The story helped them to realise that they had been making too many negative comments about their slightly overweight daughter.

Strawberry Shy didn't start out life as a shy little strawberry. Her shyness came later, once she had started to grow and change from being a tiny green berry to a middle-sized white berry. It was then that she noticed all the other strawberries in the strawberry patch were not white like her. They were slowly turning a beautiful shade of pink or red.

'There must be something wrong with me,' she thought. She then decided from this time on she would hide herself amongst the green strawberry leaves. Strawberry Shy didn't want anyone to see her.

The longer she stayed hidden, the redder all the other strawberries became, and the whiter she seemed to remain. Finally came the day of the springtime strawberry harvest. Farmer Brown walked up and down the rows of the strawberry patch, picking the ripe red strawberries. Soon her basket was filled to overflowing and the strawberry patch was empty.

Except for Strawberry Shy! She was still hiding amongst the green strawberry leaves. She was too shy to poke her head out. She watched from her hiding place as Farmer Brown carried the basket back to the farm shed, leaving Strawberry Shy all alone in the strawberry patch.

But not for long! Reaching through the fence at the edge of the strawberry patch was a branch of wild raspberries. At the end of the branch was the reddest raspberry of the whole bush. She was soaking up the springtime sun and loving every minute of its warmth and light.

Each day the branch grew longer and Raspberry Wild was carried further and further into the strawberry patch. One day she looked down to see Strawberry Shy, still hiding under a large green leaf.

'Goodness, gracious me,' said Raspberry Wild, 'Why are you hiding under a strawberry leaf?'

'I'm too shy to poke my head out – I have been hiding here because I don't have a beautiful red coat like my sisters,' whispered Strawberry Shy. 'But,' said Raspberry Wild, 'Don't you know that you need the help of the golden sunbeams to become a ripe red strawberry?' And the next minute, with a puff of wind to help her, she had knocked the leaf away from the little white berry and left her sitting in the sunlight.

After a few days in the warmth and light of the springtime sun, Strawberry Shy had lost her white coat and turned into a ripe red strawberry. She was soon as beautifully red as Raspberry Wild, although Raspberry Wild thought she was wearing a more stunning colour of red. However, before they had time to argue about it, Farmer Brown returned to the garden to look for a lost gardening glove. She saw the two red berries waiting in the sunlight and picked them both.

That night Strawberry Shy and Raspberry Wild were used to decorate Farmer Brown's birthday cake. Everyone at the party agreed they were the most beautiful red berries they had ever seen.

Pumpkin Munchkin

This story was not written intentionally for challenging introverted be-haviour. However it was a strong favourite amongst the four- to five-year-olds at pre-school and led to the idea of a school fair based on the theme of 'pumpkins' – with pumpkin stories, pumpkin games, pumpkin dolls, and a pumpkin café that sold pumpkin soup, pumpkin cakes and pumpkin scones.

Interesting feedback from one of the parents who helped organise the fair was that she had taken the Pumpkin Munchkin story as a positive theme for her family. Apparently the story helped to lift the mother out of depression. She also felt its golden theme and sense of achievement helped bring the whole family out of a despondent mood. It is therefore included in this section on shy and introverted behaviour as positive encourage-ment that the almost impossible can be achieved!

Little Munchkin lived in the wide world of open fields, where the clumps of tall bamboo creaked and swayed all day, and the long grasses by the roadside whispered pink messages to passing travellers. All through the summertime Little Munchkin was busy – busy doing her *munchkin* jobs. There was always so much to do, helping care for Mother Nature's little children. She was kept busy with butterflies whose wings were caught in spiky bushes and with lizards that had lost their tails – Little Munchkin would sew them back on again with her special mending thread. And there were always the many wildflowers that needed dewdrops brushed away so their petals could open each morning.

In the evenings Little Munchkin would wrap herself up in a leaf and fall asleep under the bright summer stars. How she loved living in the wide world of open fields, under the bright summer sky.

But Summer was coming to an end and the Autumn wind was blowing. The days were growing colder and the nights were getting longer. As the wind blew around little Munchkin, it whispered to her:

> *Autumn is here, Summer has gone,*
> *You'll need a home for the winter long.*
> *So look for a home, so warm and bright,*
> *Where a golden light shines day and night.*

'But where can I find a home so warm and bright, where a golden light shines both day and night?' Little Munchkin asked the wind.

'Follow the path of the Sun, follow the path of the Sun', whispered the wind.

So little Munchkin set off through the fields, following the path of the Sun. She hadn't gone far when she met a silver snail, who was carrying his home on his back.

'Hello Silver Snail – I'm looking for a home so warm and bright, where a golden light shines both day and night'.

'Well, well,' said Silver Snail, 'This is my home and I live here alone. There is only room here for one – keep following the path of the Sun'.

So little Munchkin kept on, following the path of the Sun through the fields. Soon she met a brown spider sitting in his web.

'Hello Brown Spider – I'm looking for a home so warm and bright, where a golden light shines both day and night'.

'Well, well,' said Brown Spider, 'This is my home and I live here alone. There is only room here for one – keep following the path of the Sun'.

So little Munchkin kept on, following the path of the Sun. Soon she came to an overgrown vegetable patch. As she climbed the rocks at the edge, she noticed a bright golden light, shining like the sun itself. She looked up and saw Great King Sunflower shining down at her.

'O Great King Sunflower, I'm looking for a home so warm and bright, where a golden light shines both day and night'.

The Sunflower King smiled, nodded his giant golden head and seemed to say,

'Look ahead, on the ground.'

Little Munchkin looked ahead, and there, sitting amongst large green leaves, was a round orange pumpkin. She was puzzled!

'Could this be my home, so warm and bright, where a golden light shines both day and night?'

Little Munchkin went up to the pumpkin, looking for a little door. She knock-knocked here, and she knock-knocked there, but she couldn't find an opening door anywhere. She walked right around the pumpkin, knocking here, and knocking there, but no matter how hard she looked, she couldn't find a little door anywhere.

By now Little Munchkin was feeling very tired, and night was on its way. She wrapped herself up in a pumpkin leaf and fell fast, fast asleep, snugly sheltered by the large wall of the pumpkin.

*

As she slept, she had a dream. She dreamt that a golden star came sailing down out of the night sky, over the swaying bamboo, across the fields and past Great King Sunflower. It landed right inside the orange pumpkin, making a star door on the top.

Next morning, when Little Munchkin woke up, she remembered her dream and climbed up to the top of the pumpkin. And there, just as in her dream, was a star door. She opened the door and peeped inside. To her delight she saw a little room glowing golden bright.

Little Munchkin was so happy. She climbed down and snuggled into her new pumpkin home, so warm and bright, where a golden light shines both day and night. And as far as I know, she is living there still.

Every morning she travels to the wide world of open fields to help care for Mother Nature's little children, and every evening she returns to her warm and snug pumpkin home. From that day to this she has always been known as 'Pumpkin Munchkin'.

The Littlest Bubble

This was written as a birthday story to help give confidence and encouragement to the smallest and shyest child in the kindergarten. It was also told one year at a Spring 'Bubble' Festival which was held in the forest on the banks of a bubbly stream. After the storytelling, children, parents and grandparents blew bubbles under the trees using different-sized bubble blowers – giant, middle-sized and tiny. The children were impressed how the smallest bubbles could so easily slip through their hands and not get popped!

This is a story about a bubble. A little bubble. In fact this bubble was the littlest bubble ever seen. This bubble could only be seen by a fairy's eye.

'It's not fair, nobody cares,' the littlest bubble whispered and sighed as it floated on down the stream with all the other bubbles. 'It's not fair that I'm so small, it's just not fair, at all, at all. Look at my great big bubble brothers. Look at their beautiful rainbow dreams. My rainbow dream can hardly be seen.'

For a long time the bubbles floated on down the country stream – the big rainbow bubbles and the one sad littlest bubble – leaving their bubbly waterfall 'mother' far behind. They floated past green willows and grass rushes, past large brown cows drinking from the sloping banks, past dark platypus burrows and rabbit furrows, around hills and through valleys.

They floated on and on, until they came to the edge of a wide green field. Here laughter and voices could be heard where happy children were picnicking under the shade of a spreading tree.

'Look!' cried one little boy, 'Bubbles, let's catch them.'

'Bubbles!' cried all the children, and they jumped up and ran to the edge of the stream. 'Bubbles, bubbles, the most beautiful bubbles we've ever seen, Bubbles, bubbles, let's catch a rainbow dream.'

Some children waded into the water, some children lay down on the bank and reached out far. All were enjoying catching the bubbles, catching their rainbow dreams. And soon all the beautiful big bubbles were gone. They were nothing more than a wish in the children's hands, nothing more than a rainbow for the children to take to dream land.

But what about the littlest bubble? The children hadn't seen him, the children hadn't caught his rainbow dream. And suddenly there he was, all alone, floating on down the stream.

'Why' he thought, 'because I'm so little I didn't get caught.'

On and on he floated, now feeling happy and brave. On and on, until the stream met the sea. There the waves took this littlest bubble far, far out into the misty blue, far, far out to where the sea fairies danced and played.

One sea fairy was busy stirring a pot of pearl when the littlest bubble floated by, the littlest bubble that could only be seen by a fairy's eye. His littlest rainbow dream caught the sea fairy's eye.

'Just what I need to colour my pot of pearl,' she said. She picked him up and popped him in her pot. And with a this-away whirl and a that-away swirl, the littlest bubble helped to make a beautiful pot of rainbow pearl.

18

Teasing or Bullying

Princess Light

This story was written for an eight-year-old girl who was suffering from low self-esteem. She was in a class of mostly girls, many of whom were cleverer and more beautiful than she was, and their teasing was starting to affect her everyday life. This was a marked contrast to her time two years before in kindergarten when she was one of the happiest and most popular children, and a child known throughout the school for her wonderful smile.

The child's favourite animal, the dolphin, was used in the story as the wise helper. 'Princess Light' was made into a picture book by the girl's older brother and sister and given as a Christmas present. The girl loved her new story and asked for it again and again. The story, and the making of the book, also helped clarify the family's awareness of the youngest child's predicament.

There was once a princess who lived in a grand castle in the forest with a beautiful garden all around. There were flowers and birds in her garden of every rainbow colour, and she had kittens and ponies and many friends to play with.

This princess was known far and wide for her beautiful smile. She had a family who loved her very much, and who knew that her smile was so beautiful because it was coming from her inner, shining light. They used to call her *Princess Light* and when she played and danced in the garden, even the flowers turned their heads towards her, thinking it was the sun itself that was smiling so brightly.

As Princess Light grew older, she began to travel to visit other parts of her land. Her favourite friend was a princess who lived in a castle in the sand dunes by the sea, and Princess Light loved to spend time there in the summer months, playing and dancing on the beach and swimming with the dolphins in the clear blue water.

For many years the two princesses had a happy friendship. But as time passed Princess Light began to notice that her friend, who was called Princess Clever, seemed to do so many things better than she could. When they were running together, her friend could run faster; when they were drawing together, her friend could draw more beautiful pictures; and when they were swimming in the sea, her friend could swim much better and faster than she could.

The more Princess Light thought about this, the sadder she became. Sometimes it even made her cross, and when she was sad *and* cross, it was not so easy for her inner light to help her smile. And when Princess Light couldn't smile, she wasn't good for anything. She couldn't run or swim or draw or do anything if she wasn't able to smile and feel happy about herself.

One day, when Princess Light was visiting Princess Clever, it was very hot, so they decided to go for a swim in the cool blue sea. They drifted far out, over the reef and into the deep ocean, where the dolphins danced and played. The two princesses had a wonderful time all morning playing with their dolphin friends. But when it was time to go back to shore, Princess Clever called out, 'Lets race.' She then swam so fast ahead that she left Princess Light all by herself in the deep waters.

Princess Light felt sad and cross that her friend seemed to be so much cleverer and faster than she was. And the sadder she became and the crosser she became, the slower she swam, until her legs and arms just stopped working altogether. Then something terrible happened, for as she stopped moving in the water, she started to sink down.

Down, down, down she went, away from the sunny clear waters of the ocean surface and down to the dark murky waters of the ocean bottom. Down, down, down, she went, until she could feel hard cold rocks under her and all around her, and she found herself trapped in a deep dark hole. She couldn't see to the right of her, she couldn't see to the left of her, and she couldn't see above her.

Then she heard a noise, and saw the silver flash of a tail. It was one of her dolphin friends who must have been following her all this time. 'Hold on to my tail,' whispered the dolphin, 'and I will try to take you back to the top. But you must kick your legs and help me, or we will not reach there together!'

So Princess Light took hold of the dolphin's silver tail and started to slowly move her legs, backwards and forwards, backwards and forwards, until she could feel herself rising out of the dark rocky hole. Faster and faster she kicked, and up, up, up she travelled, up, up, up towards the clear waters of the ocean surface. And as she burst up through the water and out into the sunshine, she took the biggest breath and then gave her dolphin friend the most beautiful smile that she had ever smiled.

'Climb on my back,' said the Silver Dolphin, who was so happy to see the princess smiling once again. 'Climb on and hold tight and we will ride the waves back over the reef.' And so Princess Light climbed onto the dolphin's back and had the ride of her lifetime all the way back to shore. Princess Clever was waiting on the beach. She couldn't believe it when she saw her friend riding on the dolphin's back across the lagoon!

When the Silver Dolphin delivered Princess Light safely to shore, he whispered to her a special message:

When you are sad or cross, don't despair and don't hide,
You have a shining light – deep inside.
This light inside will help you smile,
And your beautiful smile will shine the way,
Through darkest night and cloudy day.

For the rest of the holiday by the sea, Princess Light played happily with her friend. She never saw the Silver Dolphin again, but whenever she felt that Princess Clever was running or drawing or swimming better than she was, she remembered the special message. This helped her to keep smiling a beautiful smile and just simply trying her best!

When summer came to an end, Princess Light returned to her family in the castle in the forest. She kept her special message from the Silver Dolphin all to herself, and it always helped her through difficult times. As she grew older, she continued to play and dance in the castle garden, and the flowers still turned their heads towards her, thinking it was the sun itself that was smiling so brightly.

The Feather from the Lake

A Kikuyu Story from East Africa suitable for age five and older. This is an empowering wisdom tale for victims of teasing and ridicule. It is included by permission from the author, Catherine Karu.

Once upon a time, there lived a chief called Muugi. He had one daughter called Mweru. Mweru was as beautiful as the new moon and was loved by all who knew her.

Near chief Muugi's house was a great lake with water as clear as crystal. This lake was so special because a wonderful feather rose up out of the middle of its clear waters.

One day the chief declared, 'Whoever wants to marry my daughter must bring the feather from the lake'. Many men tried but they all failed. The water was too deep and the feather too far to reach.

There was a certain man called Giako in the chief's village but he was very poor. Everyone despised him and laughed at him for his poverty. Giako heard about the chief's promise and at once he decided to try his luck. His mother tried to dissuade him, saying, 'We are poor people. How could you be the one to marry Mweru?'

However, in spite of the warning from his mother, Giako knew that he must at least have a try. He went to the chief and bowed before him, 'Dear chief, I have come to propose marriage to your daughter'.

'Ah' said the chief, 'you must bring the feather from the lake before we talk of marriage.' And with that the chief left the court.

So Giako set off towards the lake. When he reached the lakeshore the sun was almost setting. He started slowly wading into the water and as he swam towards the feather, he sang:

Beautiful feather from the lake, please come to me, Come to me.

He moved on until the water covered his waist, and then his chest, then his shoulders and his neck. He sang again:

Beautiful feather from the lake, please come to me, Come to me.

Slowly the feather began to move in his direction. The more he sang the more the feather moved towards him. Finally he was close enough to take hold of the feather. He turned to swim back to the shore, singing as he crossed the clear waters with the beautiful feather held high in his hands:

Beautiful feather, beautiful feather, I am taking you to the dear chief.

As he reached the lakeshore he heard some noise from behind. Turning around, Giako saw a herd of cows, a tribe of goats, a flock of sheep and a flight of birds following him from the lake. 'Oh,' thought Giako, 'If all this is mine, then I am indeed the one to marry Mweru.'

When the chief saw Giako with the feather in his hands and all the animals and birds following behind, he called the elders to him. A great council was held in the village.

The next day the wedding was conducted and Giako and Mweru were married and lived happily ever after.

The Invisible Hunter

An American Indian folktale re-written by the author. This is one of my favourite versions of the classic 'Cinderella' fairytale, and an excellent 'bullying/victim' story for six- to eight-year-olds.

Long, long ago, on the edge of an Indian village, by the shores of a wide bay, there lived an old Indian warrior whose wife had long since died. He shared his wigwam tent with his three daughters, who had the tasks of cooking and cleaning and dressing the skins while he was out all day hunting.

The two older daughters were proud and lazy and considered themselves above such work. While their father was away they would beat and bully and push their youngest sister around, and make her do all the jobs.

The father had called his youngest daughter Little Rising Sun, but she was not joyful any more like the rising sun. She was thin and sad-eyed, and was often so tired from working from dawn to dark that she fell asleep from sheer weariness. Sometimes she would fall asleep over the fire and her face was scarred from the hot cinders. Her long black hair looked dull from the ashes, not shining and sleek like that of her sisters. And since there never seemed to be enough skins from the father's hunting to clothe the whole family, Little Rising Sun had only scraps to wrap about her.

One evening, when the father came home, he gathered his daughters by the fire, as he had a special story to tell them. It was about Te-Am, the Invisible One, who lived in a hunting lodge at the far end of the village with his mother. Because he was such a mighty warrior and hunter, Te-Am had been given the special power of being invisible by a great 'Chinu'. It was because of this power that none of the maidens in the village had ever seen him, although he was said to be very handsome, and his lodge was always well provided with food and soft furs.

The father continued his story: 'The mother of Te-Am, the Invisible One, has announced that Te-Am wishes to be married. He will take as his wife the first maiden who can truly see him. Many maidens have already come to his lodge, but none have been able to see him. Now you, my daughters, may have your turn.'

The two older sisters were very excited and stayed up way into the night talking about this news and what they would wear. The next morning the eldest sister dressed herself in her best robes with strings of shells around her neck and walked through the village to the great lodge of Te-Am, the Invisible One.

Te-Am's mother was waiting at the door to greet her, and said:

'My son, Te-Am the Invisible One, is out hunting. If we walk together by the shores of the lake we will soon meet him as he comes over the hills.'

So the eldest sister set out walking with Te-Am's mother, who carried a small drum with her. They hadn't walked very far when Te-Am's mother started to sing and play on the drum:

The hunter is coming, over the hills he comes,
The great hunter comes now, do you see him, do you see him?

The eldest sister looked ahead and although she could not see anyone she pretended she could. 'Yes, yes, I can see him,' she answered.

'If you can truly see him' said Te-Am's mother, 'of what is his great hunting bow made?'

'It is made from the wood of the birch tree' said the eldest sister, and from the girl's answer, Te-Am's mother knew that she had not seen her son.

Then Te-Am came closer and handed his hunting bag to his mother. The eldest sister could see the hunting bag once it was in the mother's hands, but she could not see Te-Am, and she knew she had failed her task. She sadly turned and walked back to the village.

The next morning the second sister dressed herself in her best robes with strings of shells around her neck and walked through the village to the great lodge of Te-Am, the Invisible One.

Te-Am's mother was waiting at the door to greet her, and said: 'My son, Te-Am the Invisible One, is out hunting. If we walk together by the shores of the lake we will soon meet him as he comes over the hills'.

So the second sister set out walking with Te-Am's mother, who carried a small drum with her. They hadn't walked very far when Te-Am's mother started to sing and play on the drum:

The hunter is coming, over the hills he comes,
The great hunter comes now, do you see him, do you see him?

The second sister looked ahead and although she could not see anyone she pretended she could. 'Yes, yes, I can see him,' she answered.

'If you can truly see him' said Te-Am's mother, 'of what is his great hunting bow made?'

'It is made from the wood of the ash tree' said the second sister, and from the girl's answer, Te-Am's mother knew that she had not seen her son.

Then Te-Am came closer and handed his hunting bag to his mother. The second sister could see the hunting bag once it was in the mother's hands, but she could not see Te-Am, and she knew she had failed her task. She sadly turned and walked back to the village.

The next morning Little Rising Sun rose early and wrapped herself in scraps of birch bark and put her father's old moccasins on her feet. Her sisters made fun of her as she started out, but she ignored them, thinking to herself: 'Of course I shall not be able to see Te-Am, but just to meet his mother and see his hunting lodge will make me happy.'

At last she came to the great lodge of Te-Am the Invisible One.

Te-Am's mother was waiting at the door to greet her, and said: 'My son, Te-Am the Invisible One, is out hunting. If we walk together by the shores of the lake we will soon meet him as he comes over the hills.'

So Little Rising Sun set out walking with Te-Am's mother, who carried a small drum with her. They hadn't walked very far when Te-Am's mother started to sing and play on the drum:

The hunter is coming, over the hills he comes,
The great hunter comes now, do you see him, do you see him?

Little Rising Sun looked ahead, and her eyes opened in wonder. 'Yes, yes, I can see him' she whispered.

'If you can truly see him,' said Te-Am's mother, 'of what is his great hunting bow made?'

'Why, it is made from the rainbow itself!' said Little Rising Sun.

'Ah, then you do truly see my son – come, let us hurry back to the lodge and prepare for his coming.'

On returning to the lodge, Te-Am's mother filled a basin with warm water and sweet smelling oils. She bathed Little Rising Sun and washed away the ashes from her hands and face until her cheeks began to glow. Then she dressed her in a fine robe of soft white buckskin decorated with shells and beads. Finally she brushed and combed Little Rising Sun's hair until it was sleek and shiny, and plaited in ribbons and little shells.

When she was dressed and ready, Little Rising Sun was invited to sit on the mat by the fire. Scarcely was she seated when Te-Am entered the lodge and came over to her. He smiled and said: 'So we are found, are we?' Little Rising Sun smiled back. Te-Am then asked her to stay in the lodge as his wife, and his mother began to prepare the wedding feast.

Meanwhile, Little Rising Sun's father had returned from the day's hunting and was concerned that his youngest daughter was not at home. When he asked her sisters where she might be, they told him they didn't know. So he set out to search for her.

All through the village he wandered and finally came to the lodge of Te-Am, where he could hear sounds of laughter and rejoicing from within. He looked in through the doorway and at first he didn't recognise the beautiful maiden as his daughter. But when Little Rising Sun saw her father she ran to him and hugged him and told him the story of her wonderful day. He was then invited to stay for the wedding feast, and Little Rising Sun sent for her sisters to also join the celebrations. Later that evening Little Rising Sun and Te-Am were married, and together they lived a long and happy life.

The Story of Rhodopese

An Egyptian fairytale re-written by the author. This is one of the oldest versions of the classic 'Cinderella' tale. It is an excellent 'bullying/victim' story for six- to eight-year-olds. The story can be enhanced by involving the class in puppetry or drama.

Long, long ago, in a land where the green river waters flowed into the great blue sea, there lived a young maiden named Rhodopese. She was a humble servant girl who had been captured when she was a child and carried far down the river away from her home. Her master was an old man who spent most of his time sleeping the daylight away under a shady tree. Because of his lazy habits he never saw how the other servant girls in the house bullied and teased Rhodopese.

They teased her because she looked so different to them. Their hair was straight and black while hers was curly and golden brown. They all had brown eyes and she had beautiful green eyes. Their skin was dark and rough, but Rhodopese had smooth brown skin and rosy lips, causing the other girls to call her Rosy Rhodopese. The servant girls also made her work hard and shouted at her all day:

> *Wash, wash, wash the clothes;*
> *Mend, mend, mend the robes;*
> *Chase the geese and scrub the floors;*
> *Bake the bread and polish the doors.*

Rhodopese had no friends except the birds and the animals. She had trained the birds to eat from her hand and a monkey to sit on her shoulder. An old hippopotamus would slide up on the bank out of the mud to be close to her while she was washing the clothes each morning.

Every day was the same for Rhodopese. The other girls would shout at her from morning to night:

> *Wash, wash, wash the clothes;*
> *Mend, mend, mend the robes;*
> *Chase the geese and scrub the floors;*
> *Bake the bread and polish the doors.*

At the end of the day, if Rhodopese wasn't too tired, she would go back down to the river to be with her animal friends. If she had enough energy she would sing and dance for them. One evening as she was twirling around lighter than air with her feet barely touching the ground, the old man woke up from his sleep and watched as she danced. He greatly admired her beauty and skill and thought that one so talented should not be without shoes.

So the old man ordered Rhodopese a pair of slippers – they were guilded with rose-red gold and the soles were made of soft leather. Now the servant girls really disliked her for they were jealous of her beautiful slippers.

One day, word arrived that the king of the land was holding a grand gathering and all in the kingdom were invited. The king was looking for the most beautiful woman in the land to be his queen. Oh how Rhodopese wanted to go with the servant girls, for she knew there would be dancing, singing, and lots of wonderful food. As the servant girls prepared to leave in their finest clothes, they turned to Rhodopese and gave her more chores to do before they returned.

Then they all climbed on to the raft and sailed away down the river to the king's palace, leaving a sad Rhodopese on the bank. As she began to wash the clothes in the river she hummed a sad working song. After a while the old hippopotamus grew tired of this little song and splashed back into the river. The splashing of the water wet Rhodopese's slippers. She quickly took them, wiped off the water, and placed them in the sun to dry. As she continued with her chores the sky darkened. Looking up, she saw a falcon sweep down, snatch one of her slippers, and fly away. Rhodopese was in awe, as she knew it was a magic bird that had taken her shoe. The remaining slipper she put away in her pocket.

Meanwhile the king was sitting on his throne, looking out over all the people, and feeling very bored. He would have much preferred to be riding in his chariot. Suddenly the falcon swooped down and dropped the rose-red golden slipper in his lap. Surprised, but somehow knowing that this was a sign, he announced that all the maidens in the land must try on the slipper, and the owner of the slipper would be his queen. By the time the servant girls had arrived at the celebrations, the king had left in search of the owner of the rose gold slipper. They turned their raft around and followed the royal boat back down the river.

Rhodopese heard the sound of a gong, and trumpets blaring. Then she saw the purple silk sails of the king's royal boat. She ran and hid in the rushes and watched as the royal boat pulled into the shore and the servant girls came running from their raft to try on the shoe. When the servant girls saw the shoe they recognised it as Rhodopese's slipper. They said nothing and tried to force their feet inside.

Then the king spied Rhodopese in the rushes and asked her to try on the slipper. She slid her tiny foot into the slipper then pulled the other from her pocket and began to dance. The king, overwhelmed by her beauty and her talented dancing, asked her if she would be his queen.

The other girls cried out that she was a servant like themselves and not worthy or beautiful enough to be a king's wife. The king replied; 'She is the most beautiful of all the women in my land – her eyes are as green as the river, her hair as feathery as papyrus, and her lips the rose colour of a lotus flower.'

Rhodopese and the king were married with a celebration that lasted all day and all night and far into the next day, and they lived happily together for a very long time.

How Beetle Got Her Colours

A folktale from Brazil, rewritten by the author. This story is suitable for six-year-olds and over. It emphasises respect, and being non-judgmental, and counteracts bullying.

A long time ago, in a land far away, Beetle was just plain brown. Beetle made her way slowly through the rainforest, minding her own business and not bothering anyone.

In this same forest there lived a Rat that used to tease other small animals and insects that lived there. Rat thought she was superior to all the animals because she could move so fast. Best of all she liked to laugh at and make fun of the beetle. Rat had a gang of other small animals who followed her, and joined in with her mean jokes.

Also in this forest, high up in the treetops, there lived a parrot. This parrot was colourful and beautiful and wise. And this parrot had magical powers!

For a long time Parrot had been watching Rat being mean and rude to Beetle. Parrot now thought it was time to teach her a lesson.

Parrot went to Rat and told her he had been watching her behaviour from the treetops.

'You're always teasing and taunting Beetle and the other animals, acting as if you are better than everyone else. We should have a contest and settle things once and for all,' said Parrot. 'I will organise a race between you and Beetle. Whoever wins will get to choose a beautiful new coat, of any pattern or colour.'

Now Rat was very happy about this. It would be a chance for everyone to see how fast she was. And what an easy race this would be. She had big strong legs, and could move quickly, while the beetle could only creep along on her skinny 'stick' legs.

The next day the animals met at the big fig tree, and Parrot pointed ahead to an old stump further down the path. 'Whoever gets there first will win a new coat,' said Parrot.

Parrot called the signal and the race began. Off raced Rat, streaking ahead. As she ran along she thought about how she was going to look in her new coat, and which colours and patterns she should choose. Whenever she looked back beetle was nowhere in sight, but this didn't bother Rat. She presumed that Beetle was right back by the starting line. But when Rat reached the old stump, there was beetle, sitting on the other side of the path. 'What took you so long, Rat? I've been waiting for you.'

Rat was astounded. 'How did you get here so fast?' she shouted.

'Oh, didn't you know that I can fly?' Beetle asked quietly.

'You fly? I didn't know you could fly,' said Rat, feeling very confused.

Parrot flew down and landed on the tree stump. 'There's a lot you don't know, Rat. If you would take time to get to know the other animals, you would learn a lot. You always judge others by their appearance so you never learn about who they really are. As they say, 'Never judge a book by its cover.'

Rat went grumbling off into the forest. As for Beetle, for her prize she chose a coat of blue and green – the blue of the sky and the green of fresh leaves after the rain. And she also chose to have wings that sparkled golden like the sun when it shines on the river.

To this day, beetles have colourful coats, and rats are just plain brown or grey.

The Three Billy-Goats

A Norwegian story re-written, with rhyme and repetition, by the author. Suitable for the younger children (aged three to five) this classic tale seems an appropriate one for teasing and bullying. There is a simple message – the bully gets his just punishment and the little ones can trust in bigger and stronger family and friends for protection. I have found great therapeutic effect from dramatising this story, especially if a very shy 'victim' child can play out the big Billy-goat, and a bossy, bullying child can play out the troll (and then change parts the next day).

Once upon a time there were three Billy-goats and their name was Gruff. The first Billy-goat had a little beard and little horns. The second Billy-goat had a middle-size beard and middle-size horns. The third Billy-goat had a great big beard and great big horns.

Now the three Billy-goats wanted to get to the mountains to eat sweet mountain grass. But to do this they had to cross over a bridge, and under this bridge lived a troll. This troll had eyes as round as pewter plates and a nose as long as a rake handle, and this troll didn't like anyone coming his way!

The first Billy-goat to cross the bridge was little Billy-goat Gruff.

'Trip-trap trip-trap, over my bridge trip-trap
I hear the sound of running feet,
Someone is crossing my bridge I fear – Now whom shall I meet?
Who is it comes this way clip-clap?
Who dares to cross my bridge trip-trap?'

'It is I, little Billy-goat Gruff, and I am on my way to the mountains to eat sweet mountain grass.'

'I'm coming up to get you!' roared the troll, and he stuck his long nose up over the edge of the bridge.

'Oh please don't eat me – I am so thin my bones show through my skin. Wait until my next brother comes, he will make a much better meal for you.'

'Very well,' said the greedy troll, and he went back down to his home under the bridge. And little Billy-goat Gruff continued on his way, trip-trap trip-trap, all the way to the mountains to eat sweet mountain grass.

The next Billy-goat to cross the bridge was middle-size Billy-goat Gruff.

'Trot-trot trot-trot, over my bridge trot-trot
I hear the sound of running feet,
Someone is crossing my bridge I fear – Now whom shall I meet?
Who is it comes this way bot-clot?
Who dares to cross my bridge trot-trot?'

'It is I, middle-size Billy-goat Gruff, and I am on my way to the mountains to eat sweet mountain grass.'

'I'm coming up to get you!' roared the troll, and he stuck his long nose up over the edge of the bridge.

'Oh please don't eat me – I am so thin my bones show through my skin. Wait until my next brother comes, he will make a much better meal for you.'

'Very well,' said the greedy troll, and he went back down to his home under the bridge. And middle-size Billy-goat Gruff continued on his way, trot-trot trot-trot, all the way to the mountains to eat sweet mountain grass.

The next Billy-goat to cross the bridge was great big Billy-goat Gruff.

'Tramp-tramp tramp-tramp, over my bridge tramp-tramp
I hear the sound of running feet,
Someone is crossing my bridge I fear – Now whom shall I meet?
Who is it comes this way bamp-clamp?
Who dares to cross my bridge tramp-tramp?'

'It is I, great big Billy-goat Gruff, and I am on my way to the mountains to eat sweet mountain grass.'

'I'm coming up to get you!' roared the troll, and he stuck his long nose up over the edge of the bridge.

'Very well, come up, I'm waiting for you,' said great big Billy-goat Gruff.

So the troll climbed up on the bridge. Then, with one BUTT from his great big Billy-goat horns, the great big Billy-goat pushed the greedy troll off the bridge and down, down, down into the waters below – down to where trolls should really live, never to be seen again. And great big Billy-goat Gruff continued on his way, tramp-tramp tramp-tramp, all the way to the mountains to eat sweet mountain grass.

And do you know, the three Billy-goats ate so much that they grew so fat they could hardly walk home. And as far as I know, they are still as fat as that!

Red Truck Story

This example comes from the writings of an eight-year-old girl, who was a new child at a school and the victim of some class bullying. She was encouraged by her teacher to write a story about her first term at the school. The teacher reported that the story seemed to make quite a difference for the child in the next school term, in both her attitude towards herself and towards others. It is a wonderful example of involving an older child in using creative writing to help with her/his own problem. The 'bones' of the story are included here.

The story is about a truck that had newly arrived in a car yard and all the other vehicles were making fun of it. Then one night, under cover of darkness, the truck decided to paint itself a bright shiny red. The next day it was not recognised by any of the others as the old shabby truck, and was now treated with respect. Over time the red paint washed off in the rain, and the others realised it was really the old truck underneath. But the bullying had stopped and the truck was never given a hard time again.

19

Uncooperative

The Towel Story

The following story was written by a parent from a Creative Discipline course. It is published by permission of the author, Emily Stubbs, and important notes from the author follow the story. It was an empowering experience for this parent to discover that her burning issue (managing bath time with her three-and-a-half-year-old), shared on the first night of the course, could be resolved through her own creativity. The story was presented to the child as a simple puppet show, with the song simply chanted like a nursery rhyme.

Once, in a big linen cupboard deep within a much-loved house, amongst the well-worn, cosy towels, there nestled a newcomer. Not so long ago a pair of hands had opened the wooden cupboard filled with sheets, blankets and towels, and popped in a new blue towel. He was an excited young towel, eager to have adventures – and he wanted very much to be used.

The next day the cupboard doors opened and the mother of the house reached in and lifted out the fluffy old Grandfather towel who had been keeping the new young towel company.

The following morning, the Grandfather towel was placed back in the cupboard next to the new blue towel. The young towel eagerly asked his questions of the Grandfather: 'What did you do?'

The Grandfather answered, 'I dried a little boy from top to toe as he came out of his lovely bath. I dried his face, his arms, his fingers and toes, his back, under his chin …so many places, till he was all dry and ready to snuggle into his clothes.'

The blue towel squeezed with excitement, 'It sounds wonderful, Grandfather. Such a lot for a towel to do. Do you ever forget what it is that a towel must do?'

'Oh no,' said Grandfather, 'I sing a little song that has always helped me to remember. I could sing it for you. Would you like that?'

'Oh, yes please,' said the new blue towel. So the Grandfather towel began:

Humpty diddily impty I,
Wrap him up and start to dry, first the face and then the hair,
Have to pat dry everywhere; under the arms, front and behind,
Is there anywhere else to find?
Yes – the legs, the feet, the toes; and last of all, his little nose!

The new towel was delighted with the song and asked the Grandfather towel to help him learn it.

The next day the cupboard doors opened again, and once more Grandfather towel was lifted out of the cupboard. The new towel watched him leave with a mixture of excitement and disappointment. He wanted to be used!

The following morning Grandfather towel returned. The new towel jumped up to greet him. 'How was it?' he asked.

'Delightful,' chuckled old Grandfather.

'I want a turn, I want a turn,' pleaded the new towel. 'But I'm worried that I'll forget what to do!'

'Oh no', said Grandfather towel. 'You'll be fine. You're a splendid towel, very soft. You won't forget if you sing the rhyme. Let's practise now.' Together Grandfather towel and the new blue towel sang:

Humpty diddily impty I,
Wrap him up and start to dry, first the face and then the hair,
Have to pat dry everywhere; under the arms, front and behind,
Is there anywhere else to find?
Yes – the legs, the feet, the toes; and last of all, his little nose!

The next day came and a little boy stood by his mother as she opened the cupboard doors. 'Mama,' he said, 'I haven't seen that blue towel before. May I please use it after my bath?'

'Of course,' his mother said, 'It's a new towel just waiting to be used.'

The new blue towel squealed as it was lifted out of the cupboard! Then he waited patiently on the towel rack as the boy enjoyed his bath. As the boy stepped out the towel was brought to him. The towel began to sing:

> *Humpty diddily empty I,*
> *Wrap him up and start to dry, first the face and then the hair,*
> *Have to pat dry everywhere; under the arms, front and behind,*
> *Is there anywhere else to find?*
> *Yes – the legs, the feet, the toes; and last of all, his little nose!*

After this, the blue towel wasn't brand new any more. And he was so happy to be used. As he was so fluffy and snugly the little boy asked to use him the next night. The blue towel practised again and again the little towel song, and never forgot what a towel must do!

Notes from the author:

'The Towel Story' was written specifically to address my child's aversion to being dried after showers or baths. The aversion seemed to stem from a deeper fear. My daughter had cried, even wailed, at being dried from only a few weeks old. The older and more mobile she got, she became more vocal and would scream as if murdered and run off and refuse to be dried. No amount of cajoling or reasoning seemed to remedy the situation – she always had to be restrained to be dried.

My daughter knew I'd been working on a story. The first time she heard it she was extremely attentive. She asked for it night after night for about a week, and asked for us to sing her the 'drying' song after her bath. She was so absorbed in the lyrics and locating the parts of her body that the resistance melted.

My daughter and my husband now know the song well. She loves the rhyme. The repetition of rhyming words has had a big effect on her. I found that as long as I sang or spoke in rhyme I could encourage her to cooperate with almost anything … eat her dinner, brush her hair, etc. The form and structure of language became an integral part of her 'diet'.

Now that she is four she is rhyming words as much as possible and she makes up other songs and games as she is dried / dries herself / does other things.

I think the story was a great support for my daughter, and it created a more positive focus for my husband and myself. It gave us something to work towards, rather than feeding each other's own frustrations and fears for her.

The Doves and the Hunter

A traditional Indian tale with the co-operative theme of 'strength in numbers'. Suitable for age six and older, this story could be used in the primary grades as a springboard for discussion.

One morning a flock of doves was flying across the land in search of food. Suddenly the leader of the doves saw some white grains of rice scattered on the ground under a banyan tree. He flew down towards the rice, with his flock following behind. Overjoyed at their good luck, they alighted on the ground.

The hungry doves started picking the grains, but within minutes they found their feet trapped in a net spread by a hunter. The next moment, they looked up from their trap and saw the hunter coming towards them. He was carrying a big club in his hand. The doves were sure that their moments were numbered.

But the leader of the doves was very wise and very brave. He spoke to his flock. 'Listen to me, my fellow doves. We are surely in serious trouble, but we need not lose hope. I have an idea. We can still get away unharmed if we all fly upwards together, carrying the net with us. We are small creatures and separately we can do little. But together we can easily lift the net and fly away with it.'

The doves were not sure about this idea but in fact they had no choice. So each one picked up a part of the net with their beak. Then they all flapped their wings and rose together away from the tree and high into the air. The hunter watched helplessly as the doves made their escape.

When they had flown a safe distance, the leader said to the rest of the doves, 'Half our troubles are over. But we are still not out of danger. We cannot pull our feet out of the net. I have a friend, a little mouse, who lives in a hole at the foot of the next hill. Perhaps he can gnaw at the net with his sharp little teeth and set us free.'

The doves welcomed yet another good idea from their leader, and off they flew to the place where the mouse lived. They landed on the ground in front of the mouse's home. 'What is the matter, my friend? You look worried,' the little mouse enquired of the doves' leader. 'Can I help you in any way?'

'As you can see, we have been caught in this net,' said the leader. 'We have managed to fly together and bring it so far. Can you please help us now and set us free?' 'You are most welcome,' said the mouse and soon got down to doing his work. With his sharp teeth he slowly chewed the cords of the net to pieces. One by one, all the doves were set free.

The doves thanked the mouse for his help. They also thanked their leader for saving them from an almost certain death. They were proud of such a wise dove who had taught them how to face problems by being united in strength. With a song of joy in their hearts, they flew up together across the open blue sky.

Benjie and the Turnip

The idea for this story is taken from 'Hugin and the Turnip' in The Seven-Year-Old Wonder Book *by Isabel Wyatt. It is re-written in a shorter and more simplified form by the author. It has a wonderful theme of cooperation and is suitable for age four and over.*

Once upon a time there was a little boy called Benjie, and Benjie wanted more than anything else in the whole world to have a turnip lantern for midwinter festival time. So Benjie went into the garden and planted a turnip seed, and Benjie said to the turnip:

> *Turnip, turnip, grow for me, grow as big as big can be,*
> *That I may make for midwinter time,*
> *the finest lantern that ever did shine –*
> *I want to put a candle in my turnip!*

The sun shone down on the turnip seed and the rain watered the turnip seed, and the turnip started to grow. It GREW and it GREW and it GREW until it was the biggest, roundest, juiciest turnip that anyone had ever seen. Finally Benjie decided it was time to pull up his turnip. He went into the garden and took hold of the turnip top and started to pull... and he pulled and he pulled... but the turnip did not budge one inch!

Just then, into the garden came Mother. 'What are you doing Benjie?'

I'm trying to pull up a turnip:
Mother, Mother, pull with me, pull as hard as hard can be!

So Mother took hold of Benjie, and Benjie took hold of the turnip... and they pulled and they pulled... but the turnip did not budge one inch! Just then, into the garden came Grandfather. 'What are you doing Benjie?'

I'm trying to pull up a turnip:
Grandfather, Grandfather, pull with me, pull as hard as hard can be!

So Grandfather took hold of Mother, and Mother took hold of Benjie, and Benjie took hold of the turnip... and they pulled and they pulled... but the turnip did not budge one inch! Just then, into the garden came Rabbit. 'What are you doing Benjie?'

I'm trying to pull up a turnip:
Rabbit, Rabbit, pull with me, pull as hard as hard can be!

So Rabbit took hold of Grandfather, and Grandfather took hold of Mother, and Mother took hold of Benjie, and Benjie took hold of the turnip... and they pulled and they pulled... but the turnip did not budge one inch! Just then, into the garden came Mouse. 'What are you doing Benjie?'

I'm trying to pull up a turnip:
Mouse, Mouse, pull with me, pull as hard as hard can be!

So Mouse took hold of Rabbit, and Rabbit took hold of Grandfather, and Grandfather took hold of Mother, and Mother took hold of Benjie, and Benjie took hold of the turnip... and they pulled and they pulled... but the turnip did not budge one inch!

Just then, into the garden came Caterpillar. 'What are you doing Benjie?'

'I'm trying to pull up a turnip.'

'But,' said Caterpillar, 'Don't you know the *right* way to pull up a turnip! Have you first asked the Root Gnome if you may pull it up?'

Well, Benjie hadn't thought of asking the Root Gnome. So he bent down to the ground and called out:

Gnome, Gnome, good Root Gnome,
May I take your turnip home,
That I may make for midwinter time
The finest lantern that ever did shine –
I want to put a candle in your turnip!

Then suddenly, from out of the ground next to the turnip, popped the tiniest little man.

'Goodness gracious me Benjie' said the Root Gnome, 'why didn't you say so in the first place. All this time I've been pulling and pulling and pulling the *other* way, when really there is nothing a Root Gnome likes better than to have a candle put in his turnip. Now that you have asked me, pull again.' And he popped his little head back down into the ground and disappeared.

So Caterpillar took hold of Mouse, Mouse took hold of Rabbit, Rabbit took hold of Grandfather, Grandfather took hold of Mother, Mother took hold of Benjie, and Benjie took hold of the turnip – and they pulled, and they pulled, and they pulled! Then suddenly Mouse sat down with a 'bang' on top of Caterpillar, and Rabbit sat down with a 'bang' on top of Mouse, and Grandfather sat down with a 'bang' on top of Mother, and Benjie sat down with a 'bang' on top of Mother – and in Benjie's hands was the biggest, roundest, juiciest turnip that anyone had ever seen!

Then Benjie stood up and said 'Sorry' to Mother, and Mother stood up and said 'Sorry' to Grandfather, and Grandfather stood up and said 'Sorry' to Rabbit, and Rabbit stood up and said 'Sorry' to Mouse, and Mouse stood up and said 'Sorry' to a rather squashed little Caterpillar! But really, no one was very hurt, and they all laughed a lot, and Benjie took his turnip home and 'put a candle in it'!

(And Benjie helped his mother make turnip soup from the middle of the turnip.)

20

Wild or Restless

Restless Red Pony

This story was written for a four-year-old boy who was exhibiting wild behaviour in the childcare environment. He would run around kicking and hitting other children and find it hard to keep still. The teaching staff felt he needed one-to-one supervision for the safety of the group.

This boy's favourite thing was horses, and he really soaked up the story. The teacher used it many times and always finished it with a game that encouraged the children one by one to take their place in the centre of the circle to be stroked and brushed by all the others – just like the pony!

The story has a general use for parents and teachers of four- to six-year-olds who are boisterous and restless.

There was once a little red pony,

> *Galloping galloping galloping hey, galloping galloping galloping ho,*
> *This little red pony loved to run wildly in the fields all the day,*
> *Galloping galloping galloping ho, galloping galloping galloping hey.*

Each morning in his stable he would jump and snort and kick his legs high. This little red pony didn't like to be kept inside. The farmer would bring him some fresh hay for his breakfast, but even when he was eating he could not stop jumping and kicking. Finally the farmer would open the stable door and let him run outside.

Once out in the fields he could run wild all the day,

> *Galloping galloping galloping ho, galloping galloping galloping hey.*

Most of the year the little red pony loved to be outside. But through the hot summer days the grass in the fields was brown and the dust made him itchy and uncomfortable. All through the hot summer nights he would find it hard to sleep as his coat was so hot and itchy. He would wriggle and roll and jump and kick and make such a lot of noise. The other ponies started to complain about what a disturbance he was. 'If only the little red pony knew how to keep still, if only the little red pony knew how to sleep!' they would say to each other.

Finally, help came from a most unusual friend – the grooming brush that lived on the stable shelf. This was the brush that the farmer used to groom his ponies in their stables at the end of each day. The brush knew that the farmer really wanted to brush and care for the little red pony, just like all the other ponies. But the farmer didn't want to go near this little pony's stable as he was always kicking and jumping much too wildly.

One night the brush decided to talk to the little red pony about this. He leaned out from the edge of the stable shelf and whispered:

> *Little red pony, listen well, I have a special secret to tell,*
> *If you can stand still at the end of the day,*
> *the farmer will brush your cares away.*

At first the little red pony was making so much noise with his kicking and wriggling that he didn't hear the secret. So the grooming brush called out louder:

> *Little red pony, listen well, I have a special secret to tell,*
> *If you can stand still at the end of the day,*
> *the farmer will brush your cares away.*

This time the pony heard the secret, and was very excited to be told this news. He also wanted to get some sleep each night. At the end of the next day, he came in early from the fields and tried very hard to keep still in the stable. It was very difficult to keep all four legs from moving. They loved so much to jump and kick and run. Many times he had to say to his legs – 'Please be still, please be still!'

Soon he could hear the farmer coming past his stable. What a surprise for the farmer when he found the little red pony standing so still. The farmer straight away set to work with the grooming brush – brushing the pony's back and neck and legs. Brushing this way, brushing that way. Oh it felt so good – the little red pony loved every moment of it.

After the brushing had finished all the itching had gone from the little red pony's coat. That night he was able to have the best night's sleep that he had ever had. The other ponies in the stable were delighted that the little red pony was so quiet through the night. They thanked the grooming brush for sharing his secret.

From that time onwards the little red pony always came in early from his running in the fields. He waited quietly till the farmer came and brushed his coat till it felt so, so good. He was a much happier pony now, and every evening he was able to have the best night's sleep. And he could still run wildly in the fields most of the day –

Galloping galloping galloping ho, galloping galloping galloping hey.

Of course the grooming brush was delighted as well, for there is nothing that a grooming brush likes better than to brush and care for all the ponies in the stable.

The Snail and the Pumpkin

Using a little shell for a snail, and a pumpkin sitting in the middle of an earth-coloured cloth, this story is best performed as a puppet show. It has a therapeutic quality because it is slow and simple, and can create quite a soothing mood. I have told this to three- and four-year-olds, and have often observed children taking the careful movements of the snail into their creative playtime.

[Singing] *Slowly, slowly, oh so slow, This is how a snail does go!*

There was once a little snail,
Travelling down a grassy track
She moved oh so very slowly,
Because her house was on her back.

She came across a pumpkin
Of a size so grand
And thought, here's the biggest mountain
In the whole of my land!

Moving oh so very slow,
She started up the side,
The hard work in climbing
She managed to hide.

For as she climbed she sang a song
To help the hours seem not so long

> [Singing] *Slowly, slowly, oh so slow, This is how a snail does go!*

When she reached the top she stopped for a rest
Then moved across, singing her best

> [Singing] *Slowly, slowly, oh so slow, This is how a snail does go!*

She started down the other side
If she was tired, this she did hide
She kept on singing as she went down
Until she was back on level ground

> [Singing] *Slowly, slowly, oh so slow, This is how a snail does go!*

Back on the ground, she continued on her way –
Along the grassy track, with her house on her back,
Singing a song as she travelled along.

> [Sing song several times at end]

The Grass Star Man

This story is a light-hearted tale about restlessness and transformation. It was written for a time in Australia in the early summer when grass stars (tumbleweeds) are blown down from the sand dunes and along the beaches, sometimes hundreds of them together. The story, with its repetition and sequencing, can easily be used for ages three to five, and also enjoyed by six- to eight-year-olds (and adults!).

There was once a little old woman who was walking through the sand dunes where the grasses grew thick and tall. She saw in the middle of a clump of grass something that looked like a round grassy ball. When she reached down to pick it up, all of a sudden out popped a little grass head, some grass arms and some grass legs, and a little grass star man rolled out of her hands and along the beach.

'Stop, little grass star man, I want to play with you,' cried the little old woman. But the grass star man called back:

> *Play, play – no, not I, I'm on my way back up to the sky,*
> *I've no time to play for fun, I belong back up with the sun –*
> *Run, run, run as fast as you can, you can't catch me –*
> *I'm the grass star man!*

And he continued rolling along the sand – roly-poly, tumble-bumble, over and over, with the little old woman running after him.

Soon he came to where a dog was running round and round in circles, chasing his tail. When the dog saw the grass star man he called out:

'Stop, little grass star man, I want to play with you.' But the grass star man called back:

> *Play, play – no, not I, I'm on my way back up to the sky,*
> *I've no time to play for fun, I belong back up with the sun –*
> *I've run away from a little old woman,*
> *and I can run away from you I can, I can*
> *Run, run, run as fast as you can, you can't catch me –*
> *I'm the grass star man!*

And he continued rolling along the sand – roly-poly, tumble-bumble, over and over, with the little old woman and the dog running after him.

Soon he came to where a crab was just coming out of his hole in the sand. When the crab saw the grass star man he called out:

'Stop, little grass star man, I want to play with you'

But the grass star man called back:

> *Play, play – no, not I, I'm on my way back up to the sky,*
> *I've no time to play for fun, I belong back up with the sun –*
> *I've run away from a little old woman, and a dog,*
> *and I can run away from you I can, I can*

Run, run, run as fast as you can, you can't catch me –
I'm the grass star man!

And he continued rolling along the sand – roly-poly, tumble-bumble, over and over, with the little old woman, the dog and the crab running after him.

Soon he came to where some fisherfolk were fishing by the shore. When the fisherfolk saw the grass star man they called out:

'Stop, little grass star man, we want to play with you'

But the grass star man called back:

Play, play – no, not I, I'm on my way back up to the sky,
I've no time to play for fun, I belong back up with the sun –
I've run away from a little old woman, a dog and a crab,
and I can run away from you I can, I can
Run, run, run as fast as you can, you can't catch me –
I'm the grass star man!

And he continued rolling along the sand – roly-poly, tumble-bumble, over and over, with the little old woman, the dog, the crab and the fisherfolk running after him.

Now just at that moment Father Sun poked his golden head through a window in the clouds and sent his golden sunbeams dancing down across the sky and along the sand. One golden sunbeam danced right over the top of the little grass star man and sprinkled golden sun glitter all over him.

The grass star man stopped rolling along and sat down to admire his beautiful new golden coat. 'Why,' he thought proudly, 'I must be so important that I don't have to visit the Sun – the Sun has come to visit me!'

As he sat, proudly admiring his golden coat, the little old woman caught up with him. 'Would you like to come with me?' said the little old woman. 'I'd like to hang you in my house as a Christmas Light, on Christmas Night.'

'Oh yes', said the grass star man, 'I'd like to come – With my new golden coat I'll shine as brightly as the sun.'

The little old woman took a piece of string out of her pocket, tied one end around her finger and the other end around the grass star man's golden coat, and carried him all the way back to her home. And because he now shone so golden bright, she hung him in her room as a Christmas Light.

As for the dog – he went back to chasing his tail. The crab crawled all the way back to his hole in the sand, climbed inside and fell fast asleep. And the fisherfolk... well, if you go down to the beach you might see them fishing there still, on the edge of the shore.

Jaden and the Fairy Eggs

This story grew out of the Knocking-Door-Tree poem (see Chapter Three) that I used in my first year of teaching to calm a group of children who loved to shout and run wildly through the forest on our school nature walks. It soon became a 'tradition' for the children to gather round the Knocking-Door-Tree at the beginning of the forest path and knock politely to enter, and then tiptoe quietly into the forest, with all senses awake to what they might see or hear. Both the poem and story had a great impact on changing the mood of the children on our forest walks from wild and restless to calm and quiet.

Jaden lived in a little town at the end of a winding road. Next to his house was a park and at the edge of the park was a forest. The forest was his favourite playing place. He called it the Knocking-Door-Tree forest because, right by the edge of the forest path, was a Knocking-Door-Tree. 'The forest gatekeeper must live here' he thought, and he would always knock on the door, just to be polite, before he walked down the forest path.

There were lots of other doors on other trees in the forest, and that's where all Jaden's fairyfolk friends lived. Well, he had never actually seen them, but he knew they lived there, for he often heard them playing and laughing. Sometimes he was sure he caught a glimpse of someone dancing with the sunbeams that shone down through the leaves. And sometimes he found little fairy paths they had made, and little dancing rings in the grass under the trees. 'And,' thought Jaden, 'why else would all those trees have doors in them?'

Now Jaden was very excited at this time, because Easter was coming soon. He remembered last year waking up on Easter Sunday and going outside to find a little basket on his back doorstep, full of shiny, coloured eggs.

'I wonder what the fairyfolk children find on Easter morning' he asked his mother one day. She smiled and said 'You will only find that out if you get up earlier than they do and go and see for yourself.'

'Well,' thought Jaden, 'that's exactly what I'm going to do.' So he began to think about getting up early to visit the Knocking-Door-Tree forest on Easter Sunday. In fact he was so absorbed with this idea he forgot to be excited about finding his own Easter eggs.

Easter Friday came and Jaden was busy cooking Hot-Cross buns. He carried a plate of them to share with the neighbours who lived on either side of his house. Cooking, sharing and eating buns took up most of the day.

Easter Saturday came, and what a long waiting day it was. Then it was Easter Saturday night, and Jaden went to bed very early. 'How will I know what time the fairyfolk children get up?' he asked his mother. 'The sunbeams wake them up,' she said. 'You must be there before the sunbeams, at the first call of the kookaburras.'

Next morning, at the first call of the kookaburras, Jaden woke up and looked out of the window. It was still dark, but he quietly dressed and by the time he was crossing the park a pale morning light was filling the sky. The grass was wet with dew, and this helped him get close to the forest without making any noise. He certainly didn't want to risk waking the fairy folk children with his big noisy feet.

When he reached the Knocking-Door-Tree he stopped still and looked. Apart from seeing a few little ants already busy at their work in the grass by the door, there was nothing else. He couldn't help feeling a little disappointed. 'Maybe the fairyfolk children don't get anything for Easter? Maybe I've come too late? Or... maybe the forest gatekeeper doesn't have any children!'

This last thought encouraged him to look further. So he crept down the forest path to the tree with the next little door. There, to his surprise, was the tiniest basket he had ever seen. It was sitting right on the edge of the doorstep. He bent down and looked inside the basket and saw the tiniest eggs he had ever seen. They were even tinier than the carrot seeds he had helped his Mother plant in the garden that week.

Jaden kept walking, going from little door to little door, all along the path. Outside the next little door were three little baskets, outside the next – two, the next – none, the next – one, and so on, until he came to where the path led out of the forest on the other side. He turned and walked quietly back through – how he would have loved to have taken just one little basket to show his mother. But he knew that this could never do! Imagine how disappointed one of the fairy folk children would have been if they had woken up to find an empty front step.

And then he remembered that in his hurry to visit the Knocking-Door-Tree forest so early, he had completely forgotten to look on his own back step. He ran across the park as fast as he could, and in through his back gate. The sunbeams were shining across the grass and onto the step, and there, glistening in the morning light, was his Easter basket full of coloured eggs. He carried it inside and up onto the kitchen table, and started to unpack the eggs out of their straw nest.

When he lifted up the bottom egg, hiding in the straw was a tiny fairy basket – just like the ones he had seen in the Knocking-Door-Tree forest. And tucked into the basket, on top of the tiny eggs, was a little note:

> *Some fairy eggs filled with Easter light,*
> *For a little boy so kind and bright.*
> *In your autumn garden please do sow*
> *And come the springtime, flowers will grow.*

SECTION FOUR

STORIES FOR CHALLENGING SITUATIONS

This section of the book touches on some of the difficult experiences that young children may meet in their growing years. From straightforward situations like moving house or school, to more complex ones like dealing with fear, illness and grieving, story examples are included here that may help a child cope with a new challenge. I don't claim that stories alone can heal such situations, but they can certainly help children (and parents/carers) to face their anxieties and fears with courage and imaginative solutions.

21

Change or Transition

Anything New

A story about moving to a new home or new school – this can be adjusted to suit different kinds of 'moving'. The story could be told to four-year-olds and up, and a different 'pouch' animal with a different name could be substituted for the wombat (e.g. a possum or a kangaroo).

If told to school-age children, they could get involved by illustrating and / or acting out the different scenes, and discussing how it felt for them to move to a new house or school. A creative writing exercise could follow on this theme.

Womby Woo was a little wombat who didn't like anything new.

His home was inside his mother's warm, furry pouch and this is where he wanted to stay. It was so comfortable here – why should he want to move anywhere else?

Sometimes Womby Woo would climb out to have a drink at the waterhole or nibble some sweet mossy grass, but he never stayed very long out in the world. If the wind blew around him and ruffled his fur, back into his mother's pouch he would jump.

Womby Woo didn't like anything new!

If raindrops started to fall on his head, back into his mother's pouch he would jump.

Womby Woo didn't like anything new!

If other wombats came too close to him, back into his mother's pouch he would jump.

Womby Woo didn't like anything new!

His mother's pouch was his home, the only home he had ever had. But Womby Woo was growing and his mother's pouch was staying the same size.

Early one morning, when Womby Woo had finished drinking an unusually large amount of water at the water hole and nibbled an unusually large amount of sweet, mossy grass, he tried to climb back inside his pouch home. But this time only his head seemed to fit into the pouch and his body stayed outside. He tried again, putting his tummy in first, but still his body stayed outside. He tried again, putting his feet in first, but still his body stayed outside.

What was Womby Woo to do? Suddenly he found himself out in the big wide world, where everything was new. And Womby Woo didn't like anything new!

Looking around, Womby Woo saw a large bush. He crawled underneath and made a hole in the sand and curled up inside. It wasn't the same as his mother's pouch but it was all he had. He tried to sleep but everything was too new.

Suddenly, from somewhere in the bush, came the loudest, strangest sound Womby Woo had ever heard.

'OO, OO, OO, OO, AH, AH, AH, AH, OO, OO, OO, OO, AH, AH, AH, AH'

Womby Woo looked up and on a branch right above his head was a large brown-and-white bird.

'Who are you?' said Womby Woo, 'and why are you making such a loud noise?'

'I am Mr Kookaburra and this is my laugh. And I am laughing at you, Womby Woo! OO, OO, OO, OO, AH, AH, AH, AH, OO, OO, OO, OO, AH, AH, AH, AH'

'What is so funny?' asked Womby Woo.

'OO, OO, OO, OO, AH, AH, AH, AH, You are so funny, Womby Woo. It is so funny that you don't like anything new. Don't you know that 'new' can be FUN.'

Womby Woo was very surprised to hear this. 'It is not fun lying here in a cold sandy hole' he said.

'Then follow me,' said Mr Kookaburra, and he flew out of the bush and along the track, laughing as he went, 'OO, OO, OO, OO, AH, AH, AH, AH, OO, OO, OO, OO, AH, AH, AH, AH'

Womby Woo stood up and cautiously followed Mr Kookaburra. The moon had just risen in the sky and was shining brightly over the distant hills. The wildflowers along the track were nodding their pretty heads towards him. It seemed as if they were saying 'Welcome to the world.' Dragonflies were flittering from bush to bush, and frogs were croaking all around. Womby Woo was surprised to find how beautiful the outside world could be.

The track led down to a waterhole, a new waterhole, a waterhole his mother had not yet taken him to. Around the edge, having dust baths and playing in the shallow water, were many other little wombats, just about his size. They looked up when they saw Womby Woo and called out to him – 'Come and play with us, Womby Woo.'

So Womby Woo joined the other little wombats and played all night. The next morning the mother and father wombats arrived at the waterhole to meet up with their little ones. After digging holes together in the soft ground under the trees they slept there all the next day. It was a warm, cosy feeling for Womby Woo to be surrounded by his wombat family once again.

When he woke up he couldn't wait to play with his friends. It was such FUN! And every night, Womby Woo's friends helped him to do something new and to learn something new. To his surprise, Womby Woo began to like things that were new.

He would often hear Mr Kookaburra laughing at dusk and dawn from the tall treetops, OO, OO, OO, OO, AH, AH, AH, AH, OO, OO, OO, OO, AH, AH, AH, AH.

But Womby Woo knew he wasn't laughing at him any more. Mr Kookaburra was just having FUN!

A Chameleon Story

A mother at one of my parenting courses in Nairobi asked the group to workshop a story for her six-year-old boy who was having trouble with change and transition. The boy was finding it unusually disturbing to move from one activity to another – both at home and at school – e.g. from playtime to morning tea, from outside time to story time, from bath time to bedtime, etc.

Together we worked on some ideas using a chameleon as the central character. The mother had noticed her son's fascination with the chameleons that he found from time to time in their garden. The story built an interesting connection with colour cards for different transition times.

Chameleons are unique creatures in their own right. Known for their ability to change colour, they can be seen in various shades including brown, green, blue, yellow, red, black or white. The story used these seven colours with seven chameleon-shaped colour cards for seven identified activities – playtime, tidy-up time, mealtime, jobs-time, bathtime, story-time, and bed-time. The idea of working with the cards after hearing the story made a significant difference for the boy's acceptance of transition.

The story was a simple recounting of the day in the life of a little chameleon, using the same rhythms as a day in the life of the boy. The story started off like this (I have left it open ended for individual changes depending on different family rhythms and needs):

Once upon a time there was a little chameleon who lived with his family in a hollow log at the bottom of a garden. Every day he would wake up in the morning, put his brown coat on, and eat some brown worms for breakfast. Then with his green coat on he would go outside and play on the green mossy rocks. When it was time to tidy up he would wear his …coat [etc. etc.] until night-time came and it was time to wear a black coat the colour of the black night sky (with tiny silver stars on the back).

Note: A song or rhyme for each change can add extra strength to this little tale –

> *I change my colour to help me find my way,*
> *I change my colour many times a day.*

Farmer Just Right

This story has been used by families of children aged four to seven to help give a sense of stability in times of transition. On the farm of Farmer 'Just Right' everything has its place and function. An extended version of the story was used by a mother as a humorous approach to talking her five-year-old through his habit of hiding in a cupboard and soiling his pants. On the farm of Farmer 'Just Right' the correct place for this activity was, of course, the toilet. There is also delicious mud play in this story, which could help a child who doesn't like to get dirty to take a few more risks –

the story encourages getting muddy but with the promise of being able to clean up afterwards.

There was once a little white duck who didn't like being with all the other white ducks on the pond. Instead, this little white duck loved playing in the muddy puddles at the edge of the pond. So instead of looking white, more often than not she was muddy all over. All the other ducks used to call her 'Puddy Muddles' because she so loved to play in the muddy puddles. All through the day she played in the puddles on her own. Then, when she was hungry and tired, she washed off the mud in the pond water and swam back to be with her mother. She loved to fall asleep tucked up inside her mother's soft downy feathers. The next day back she would go again, to splash and play in the muddy puddles.

The pond where all the ducks lived was on a farm belonging to Farmer Just Right. Farmer Just Right loved everything on her farm to be Just Right – 'A place for everything and everything in its place' she would sing as she went about her daily chores. It made her happy to look out of the farmhouse window and see the white ducks on the pond, the cows in the fields, the hens pecking in the yard and the pigs rolling in the mud in their pigpen.

One day when Farmer Just Right was walking by the side of the pond she looked down and saw something round and muddy playing in the muddy puddles. 'Goodness me,' said Farmer Just Right, 'one of the piglets must have climbed out of their pig pen.' Without further ado, she picked up the round muddy thing and carried it back to the pigpen. When she reached the pigpen she carefully dropped it in, singing to herself, 'A place for everything and everything in its place.' Feeling happy that she had been able to help, she continued going about her chores.

Now the round muddy thing was not a piglet at all. It was really the little white duck called 'Puddy Muddles'. At first she was quite happy to be in the pigpen as there was so much lovely mud in there. She rolled about with the other piglets who didn't seem to notice that she wasn't like them because she was so covered in mud. She rolled and played most of the day. However, when the sun went down and it started to grow dark, she wasn't so sure that this was where she wanted to be. All the other piglets had curled up around their big fat muddy mother and were going to sleep. But Puddy Muddles missed the soft feathers of her own mother and was not able to fall asleep like the others.

Puddy Muddles was also feeling very hungry as the scraps of food that the farmer had thrown into the pigpen weren't as tasty as the slugs and worms her mother used to give her for tea. So Puddy Muddles decided it was time to somehow find her way back home. She waddled to the fence of the pigpen but when she tried to climb out, because she was so slippery with mud, she kept sliding back down. Then she had to try to find a way under the fence instead. This way out needed a great deal of digging, which she was able to do with her strong duck beak.

After a long time and much hard work she eventually made a tunnel through the mud and under the fence. She emerged on the other side looking even muddier than before. Now there was mud in her ears and eyes and mouth and up her nose. Even Puddy Muddles didn't like to be covered in this much mud!

If Farmer Just Right had been looking out of her farmhouse window that evening she would have seen a round muddy thing waddling across from the pigpen and down to the pond. But Farmer Just Right was so tired from a hard day's work keeping everything on her farm Just Right and she had already fallen asleep. Puddy Muddles made her way slowly back to her pond and dived right into the cool, cleansing water. It took a very long time for her to wash off all the mud – pigpen mud seemed to be much thicker and stickier than puddle mud – but eventually she was clean and white and ready to swim back to her mother.

Mother Duck was so happy to see her little lost duck swimming in the moonlight across the pond. She had saved some special slugs and worms, so fortunately Puddy Muddles had plenty to eat. Then, without saying a word, she tucked up amongst her mother's soft feathers and fell fast asleep. And to this day Mother Duck never found out where her little duck had been, and Farmer Just Right never found out that it was not a piglet that she had returned to the pigpen.

To this day, Farmer Just Right has never found another round muddy thing in the muddy puddles on the edge of the pond. Puddy Muddles still enjoys playing in the mud but she always makes sure she stays out of the way of the farmer. And when Farmer Just Right looks out of her farmhouse window, she can always see the white ducks on the pond, the cows in the fields, the hens pecking in the yard and the pigs rolling in the mud in their pig pen. 'A place for everything and everything in its place,' she happily sings as she goes about her daily chores.

Little Shell

This story was written for three- to four-year-olds, and is best performed as a simple puppet show. It has been used with great success in playgroups to settle new children. As well as providing a warm, 'homely' theme, it has helped engage children in creative play with simple materials – for example, a basket of shells.

A little white shell was floating all alone on the blue, blue sea. It was wondering 'Where can I go, what can I be?'

All of a sudden a wave took the little shell and rolled it

Roly-poly tumble-bumble over and over ...

And it landed upside down in the water. Then another wave rolled it

Roly-poly tumble-bumble over and over ...

Before the little shell had time to wonder whether it was upside-down or right-side-up a very big wave rolled it

Roly-poly tumble-bumble over and over ...

And the wave dropped the little shell onto the dry sands of a long golden beach.

The little shell lay on the sand, pink and white and patterned bright, glistening in the morning sunlight. It wondered to itself 'Where can I go, what can I be?'

Meanwhile an old woman had set out for an early morning walk along the beach. As she walked along the sands she saw the little shell, pink and white and patterned bright. She picked it up and looked at it. 'I know a little girl who would like to play with you,' she said, and she put the little shell in her pocket and walked back home.

When she reached the house she tiptoed into the bedroom where her granddaughter lay fast asleep. The old woman put the little shell, pink and white and patterned bright, on the table next to the bed. Then she went into the kitchen to make some porridge for breakfast. The shell sat on the table and wondered to itself 'Where can I go, what can I be?'

When the granddaughter woke up she saw the beautiful shell on the table and picked it up and started to play with it. The shell made a wonderful dish for her dolls' tea party. Then the shell was turned into a little telephone for her teddy bear.

Soon grandmother called the family for breakfast. The little shell sat on the table while the girl ate her porridge. After breakfast she took the shell out onto the sand in front of the house and played and played – digging in the sand, building castles and making patterns.

Grandmother sat in her chair on the veranda watching her granddaughter playing. The little girl called out 'Thank you Grandmother – it is such a lovely toy.'

The little shell knew that at last it had found a friend and a home. It knew it was where it was meant to be, and doing what it was meant to be doing.

22

Tidy-Up Time

Tidy Teddy

A story for children (and parents) that will help encourage the tidying of toys and bedrooms. Suitable for ages four to eight. Also suitable for turning into a picture book with the child/children involved in drawing the untidy room (with the toys all jumbled up, topsy-turvy, upside-down and inside out), Tidy Teddy, the Lamp Doll and the tidy room (with the toys sorted, neatly stacked and right-side-up).

Teddy lived in the toy box in the corner of the bedroom. Many other toys also lived there, and although the box was a very long and very wide home, there were always toys spilling out onto the floor – jumbled up, topsy-turvy, upside-down and inside out.

The bedroom belonged to a little girl called Amber. Amber was not interested in tidying up her toys. It was hard to call her lazy – usually her parents just did the work for her so she never had a chance to find out what fun it could be to put her toys away. Amber's parents would come into the room almost every day and complain about the toys being jumbled up, topsy-turvy, upside-down and inside out. Then they would set to work to sort things out, so that for a little while the toys were all sorted and tidy again.

Teddy loved it when everything was sorted and tidy – it helped him feel calm and peaceful inside. But within a few hours of Amber playing in the room, things were back to their untidy state – all jumbled up, topsy-turvy, upside-down and inside out.

One day the room received an important addition that would change things forever. Amber was given a beautiful lamp for her birthday. It was not an ordinary lamp with an ordinary lamp-stand – this lamp-stand was a golden doll and the lampshade was a pink flower-patterned umbrella. The lamp was placed high up on Amber's dressing table, and from here the Lamp Doll could see all over the room.

All the toys in the room could look up from their spots on the floor or in the toy-box and see the Lamp Doll. They agreed she was very beautiful, but Teddy couldn't take his teddy-eyes off her! He had never seen such a lovely sight, especially in the evenings when the doll was all lit up, golden and bright.

However, after only a few nights of the Lamp Doll arriving in the bedroom, its light stopped working. No matter how many times Amber tried to switch it on, it just didn't work. Amber's parents checked the globe, they even called in the neighbour who knew about electrical things, but nobody could find any reason why the lamp wouldn't light up.

Teddy felt very sad, but there was nothing he could do about it. After all, he was just a toy. He looked around at the untidy mess in the room and this made him feel even worse. Amber's parents were so busy trying to work out why the lamp wasn't working, they had now stopped bothering to tidy the room.

Teddy realised he was feeling annoyed as well as sad. Why didn't Amber tidy up? Couldn't she see that a tidy room could help everyone feel a little better, calmer, happier? Then he had an interesting idea – perhaps this was the reason why the Lamp Doll had stopped working. Why would such a beautiful doll want to shine her light out over a messy room?

Teddy decided to do something about the mess. He might be just a toy, but he could try to be a tidy toy! He set to work sorting and sifting – picking up puzzle pieces, stacking books back on their shelf above the toy box, placing dolls and cars carefully into their homes and garages – generally putting things back where they belonged.

At last all the toys that had been jumbled up, topsy-turvy, upside-down and inside out were sorted, neatly stacked and right-side-up. Teddy stood back to admire his work. Just at this moment, the Lamp Doll switched herself on and shone golden light across the room. At the same time as the light came on, Teddy was sure he could hear a small whisper coming from the dressing table – 'Thank-you Tidy Teddy!' The golden doll was speaking to him!

Teddy was so happy he almost burst with joy and pride. He settled back into the toy box, lay there for a long time watching the beautiful Lamp Doll, then finally fell fast asleep. His teddy-dreams that night were the best dreams he had ever had.

Amber was also happy now that her lamp was working again, and Amber's parents were even happier to see that their daughter's room had been tidied without their help.

From this time on, Teddy took on the role of tidying up the toys. He didn't mind the extra work if it meant that the beautiful Lamp Doll would shine golden light each night across the room. As he worked he sang to himself:

I'm a tidy teddy and I love to do my best,
Picking up the toys and cleaning up the mess.

Soon Teddy noticed that Amber was taking a bit more care with her toys – perhaps she could hear his song? Soon, without even planning it, they were sharing the tidy-up tasks together.

Of course, Teddy had to be careful not to let his new role get out of hand – there were times when Amber was playing and needed her toys out of their box and off the shelf. It was not always time for tidying up. Teddy had to learn to be patient with this and soon grew to be content with a 'once-a-day' tidy-up time. As long as the toys were all sorted, neatly stacked and right-side-up each evening, the Lamp Doll continued to shine her golden light over the room.

Little Straw Broom

This story/poem was written to enthuse 'little helpers'. It has been used with all ages of children and adults – it seems to defy categorisation for just one age group. It is often told as a puppet show using three little dolls with felt hats (blue, red and yellow) to symbolise the three men. A tiny straw broom can be made from pine needles, and a house can be built from logs and/or tree roots. It has also worked effectively as a play, with felt hats for the actors, and a small broom.

Little-Man Blue Hat and Little-Man Red Hat lived together under the roots of the flame and thorn tree. But do you know that their home was the messiest home that you ever did see!

> *There were crumbs, crumbs, everywhere.*
> *There were crumbs under the table,*
> *There were crumbs under the chairs.*
> *There were crumbs all over the mat,*
> *There were crumbs under the beds,*
> *There were even crumbs under the pillows*
> *where the little men rested their heads.*

They had a little straw broom – it lived in the corner of the room. But Blue Hat and Red Hat didn't know how to use the broom properly.

The little straw broom would look out over the room and sigh – 'If only someone could use me properly, I could clean up this mess in the wink of an eye.'

Now Blue Hat and Red Hat were meant to sweep the room. But whenever it was Blue Hat's turn, Blue Hat simply couldn't be bothered. He would take hold of the little straw broom and slowly drag it round the room, singing his 'Couldn't be bothered' song:

I couldn't be bothered, I couldn't be bothered,
I couldn't be bothered to work;
All through the day, I just want to play –
the sweeping is something I shirk.

So when Blue Hat had finished, the crumbs were just as they were before.

[Repeat 'Crumbs' poem]

Whenever it was Red Hat's turn, Red Hat was always in too much of a hurry. He would take hold of the little straw broom and quickly sweep the room, singing his 'swisherty-swat' song:

Swisherty swat, swasherty swit,
the little straw broom goes that way and this,
Swasherty swit, swisherty swat,
the little straw broom goes this way and that.

And when Red Hat had finished, the crumbs were even worse than before!

[Repeat 'Crumbs' poem]

Then, one day, Little-Man Gold Hat came to stay. He walked in the door and saw the crumbs all over the floor. 'Goodness gracious me,' said Gold Hat, 'Where is the broom? I must sweep this room.'

Gold Hat went straight to the corner of the room, took hold of the little straw broom, and started to sweep, singing his 'Sweep-it-all-up' song:

Sweep it all up, sweep it all up,
Little Gold Hat can sweep it all up,
Crumbs in a pile will make him smile,
Little Gold Hat can sweep it all up.

Gold Hat swept everywhere. He swept under the tables, he swept under the chairs. He swept all over the mat, he swept under the beds. He even swept under the pillows where the little men rested their heads.

When Gold Hat had finished, the crumbs were in a pile in the middle of the room. Gold Hat put back the little straw broom, and the little straw broom was so tired it fell fast asleep.

And Gold Hat, Red Hat and Blue Hat sat down at the table and shared currant buns and tea.

Three little men had three little hats,
Three little men together –
Blue Hat, Red Hat, Golden Hat too,
Sharing a home together,
Caring for a home together.

23

Fear or Nightmares

God's Garden

I used to tell this story to my boys at times of troubled sleep and nightmares (from ages four to eight). It helped soothe them and lull them back to sleep. It uses the classic theme of the stork that brings the baby, and gives images that can help lead a frightened child back into 'the land of sweet dreams'.

Do you ever wonder where God lives? Try to picture his home, not in a house like you live in, but in a beautiful garden, a garden that God calls 'heaven'. Here the plants have leaves made of silver, silver like the moonlight on the dark sea, and their flower petals are gold, as golden as the sun. There are many different flower gardens in heaven, each on different white cloud islands, with rainbow bridges stretching their bright colours from one island to the next. There are so many beautiful things in God's garden it would be impossible to describe them all to you tonight.

But there is one thing I want to tell you about. In between the gardens of silver and golden plants runs a lively little stream, a stream not filled with drops of water like the rivers and streams down in our world. This heavenly stream is filled with thousands of tiny star-lights, bouncing and jostling and tumbling along together. The stream weaves its way into God's garden after travelling from the far corners of the night sky, collecting new little star-lights on its way. Once it reaches the centre of the garden, the centre of heaven, it tumbles over a great waterfall. All the little star-lights end up in a light pool that is already so full of sparkling star-lights that it shines as brightly as the sun – one is almost blinded by its radiant brilliance!

Now, as you can imagine, all the little star-lights that have tumbled over the waterfall feel very excited and privileged to be part of this wonderful pool of light. They remember the stories their mother stars have told them many times, about the long journey they had to take to reach this very important place, and about the great white angel birds that encircle the pool with their loving embrace. The little star-lights can see them now – standing around the edge of the pool of light, with their shining white wings spread out to touch each other, arrayed in majestic splendour. Can you picture this beautiful sight?

Not only are the little star-lights excited to be here, but they are excited at the new journey and task that lies ahead of each one of them. They know that the white angel birds are God's special messengers. The angel birds wait by the pool's edge till news is heard from far below on earth that a new baby boy or girl is to be born into the world. On hearing such news, one of the birds flies down into the pool of light and chooses a little star-light. Holding it in a silken cradle, it then sets off, up and over God's garden and across the night sky – flying on the long journey down to the earth below.

This star-light is a present from heaven that God gives to each new baby born on earth. The white angel bird, on reaching the world after its long journey from the heavenly garden, gives this wonderful present to the new baby. It places the star-light deep inside the baby's heart, and there it stays forever, warm and bright.

Here is a little prayer for the star-light given to the new born child:

> *Little star, come from far, Guide my path, be my staff,*
> *Warm and bright, like a candle light,*
> *Little star, in the darkness, be my light.*

I wonder which little star-light was chosen for you when you were born?

I think perhaps God has given us each a star-light from his pool of light in heaven because he wants to share his own garden, his own home, with all of us. So if you wonder where God lives, his home is never too far away: we all have a little part of his home right here inside us, right here on earth.

The Antelope, the Butterfly and the Chameleon

A Kikuyu Story from East Africa, included here by permission of the author, Lucy Njuguna. This is a wonderful example of a traditional African story told to children to help them face their fears of the dark and the unknown. Suitable for age five and older.

Once upon a time there lived an antelope who was always roaming in the forest. All the other animals were against him and chased him all the time. One day he decided it would be good for him to build a large house, one bigger than all the trees in the forest. When he had finished building it he divided the house into many little rooms, so that when any other animal came by he would be able to hide deep inside.

During the day, the antelope used to go and look for food and water. He also liked visiting his friends and telling them about his house. But one day, when he left his house, he forgot to close the door. Sometime later, when a butterfly was fluttering around the flowers, it found that the door was not closed. So it fluttered inside and flew to the darkest corner to rest.

When the antelope came back and found that the door was wide open he was too frightened to go inside. He asked in a loud voice, 'Who is in the house of the antelope?' and the butterfly answered:

> *Ninii Kibutabuti na Iguru, ninii Kiminja muinge*
> (I am the one who flutters up and down)

When the antelope heard this, he ran towards the forest to look for help. On the way he met an elephant. The elephant asked him, 'What have you seen Mr. Antelope? Why are you running so fast?' The antelope replied, 'There is somebody in my house and I am frightened to go inside.'

'Let's go,' said the elephant, 'I will help remove him.'

When they arrived at the antelope's house, the elephant asked in a loud voice, 'Who is in the house of the antelope?' The butterfly again answered:

Ninii Kibutabuti na Iguru, ninii Kiminja muinge

When the elephant heard this he ran away, back to the forest.

So the antelope went quickly to look for other animals to help. One by one they came to his house but, like the elephant, they were all too afraid to go inside and remove the butterfly.

When the antelope was sitting by his door, thinking what to do, he remembered that there was one more animal he had not asked. This was the chameleon. So he ran to find the chameleon in the forest.

The chameleon asked him, 'What have you seen, Mr. Antelope? Why are you running so fast?' The antelope replied, 'There is somebody in my house and I am frightened to go inside.'

'Let's go,' said the chameleon, 'I will help remove him'.

When they arrived at the antelope's house the chameleon asked in a loud voice, 'Who is in the house of the antelope?' The butterfly again answered:

Ninii Kibutabuti na Iguru, ninii Kiminja muinge

When the chameleon heard these words, he started to walk in. All the other animals were gathered around the door and they saw this and were frightened. But they waited and watched to see what would happen.

As the chameleon entered each room he kept asking the same question, 'Who is in the house of the antelope?'

Ninii Kibutabuti na Iguru, ninii Kiminja muinge, answered the butterfly many times.

Finally the chameleon reached the dark corner where the butterfly was hiding. He quickly caught it and took it back outside to show the other animals. When they saw how tiny it was, they all went back to the forest very ashamed of themselves.

From that day onwards the antelope and the chameleon were close friends.

The Elves and the Shoemaker

A well-loved fairytale, rewritten by the author. This is a story to induce hope in the 'impossible' and a trust in help from unimaginable sources. A lovely bedtime tale for age five and older.

There was once a shoemaker who lived with his wife in a little cottage at the edge of town. It happened that this shoemaker, through no fault of his own, had become so poor that he only had enough money left to buy leather to make one more pair of shoes.

That evening he went into his workshop, spread out the leather on his workbench, and cut out the pieces – ready for work the next morning. Then he and his wife went to bed.

While they were sleeping, something happened!

Pull the thread and stitch the shoe,
Pull it tight and that will do.
Fairy fingers nimble light,
First the left and then the right.

The next morning when the shoemaker awoke he went into his workshop ready to start work. There, to his surprise, sitting on his workbench, was a beautifully-made pair of shoes. He picked them up and looked at them, inside and out – what beautiful stitching, what fine work – he had never seen such perfect shoes! He put them in the window, and very soon a customer came in, paid more than the usual amount for the shoes, and took the shoes away.

Now the shoemaker had enough money to buy leather to make two more pairs of shoes. That evening he went into his workshop, spread out the leather on his workbench, and cut out the pieces – ready for work the next morning. Then he and his wife went to bed.

While they were sleeping, something happened!

Pull the thread and stitch the shoe,
Pull it tight and that will do.
Fairy fingers nimble light,
First the left and then the right.

The next morning when the shoemaker awoke he went into his workshop ready to start work. There, to his surprise, sitting on his workbench, were two beautifully-made pairs of shoes. He picked them up and looked at them, inside and out – what beautiful stitching, what fine work! He put them in the window, and very soon two customers came in, paid more than the usual amount for the shoes, and took the shoes away.

Now the shoemaker had enough money to buy leather to make four more pairs of shoes.

And so it went on – every evening the shoemaker would spread his leather out on his workbench and cut out the pieces ready for work in the morning. And every morning the shoes would be beautifully finished, waiting for him in his workshop.

One evening, when the shoemaker was busy in his workshop, his wife came to him and said: 'For a long time now someone has been visiting us in the night and doing this special work – why don't we stay up tonight and hide behind the curtains and see who it could be?'

The shoemaker thought this a very good idea. Leaving the lamp burning, the shoemaker and his wife hid behind the curtains. They watched and they waited, and they waited and they watched, and they watched and they waited, and they waited and they watched … then, at the stroke of midnight, they saw come dancing into the room two tiny little men. Not a stitch of clothing did they have on! They jumped up onto the workbench and with their tiny fairy hammers and fairy needles they set to work – hammering and stitching, stitching and hammering – all the while singing their working song.

> *Pull the thread and stitch the shoe,*
> *Pull it tight and that will do.*
> *Fairy fingers nimble light,*
> *First the left and then the right.*

All through the night the tiny men worked, until the shoes were beautifully finished, and sitting on the workbench. Then the little men jumped down and danced out of the room.

The shoemaker's wife said to her husband – 'I think we should give some gifts to these little folk who have been so kind to us – why don't we make them some clothes?'

The shoemaker thought this a very good idea. He spread out two tiny pieces of leather on his workbench, cut out the pieces and set to work, hammering and stitching, stitching and hammering, until he had finished two tiny pairs of shoes.

Meanwhile the shoemaker's wife had taken out her sewing basket and with her needle and cloth had stitched and sewed two tiny shirts and two tiny pairs of trousers. Then with her wool and knitting needles she knitted two tiny hats. When she had finished she laid out the clothes on the work-bench next to the shoes. Then, leaving the lamp burning, she and her husband hid behind the curtains. They watched and they waited, and they waited and they watched … then, at the stroke of midnight, they saw come dancing into the room the two tiny men who jumped up onto the table, ready to start work. But there was no leather waiting for them. What could these things be they wondered?

They started to try them on. They tried on the tiny shirts, and they fitted perfectly. They tried on the tiny trousers, and they fitted perfectly. They tried on the tiny shoes, and they fitted perfectly. They tried on the tiny hats, and they fitted perfectly.

> *Happy little men are we,*
> *Gaily dressed as you can see,*
> *No more shoemakers to be!*

With their new clothes on the little men sang and danced around the room. Then they danced out the door – never to be seen again. And the shoemaker and his wife, who had been kind to those who had been good to them, lived happily for the rest of their lives.

The Sky's Blue Cloak

Given as a 6th birthday gift (handwritten on the back of a beautiful sky-blue painting) this story was written for one of my boys to help with his fear of the dark. It is reprinted here by permission of the writer, Susan Haris. Though drawing on a Christian theme, the story has a beautiful message that transcends all religions.

A very long time ago, in the middle of a freezing cold night, Baby Jesus was born in a far away land in a little town called Bethlehem. Mother Mary was dressed in a beautiful red gown and over her head and shoulders she wore a deep blue mantle. She wrapped her baby in the folds of her cloak, and held him safe and warm in her arms.

It was a clear night, with many twinkling silver stars. Above the place where the Christ Child was born, the sky was lit by a wonderful, bright golden star. From that night onwards, whenever her baby was frightened or upset, Mother Mary would take him in her arms, wrap her deep blue cloak around him, and carry him out to look up at the beautiful stars shining in the dark night sky.

The weeks and months passed, and one day, when the little Christ Child was playing in the garden with a friend, suddenly a loud storm broke the sky. There was clapping of thunder and flashing of lightning, and the two boys were terrified. Trembling with fear, they ran inside to find Mother Mary, who gently enfolded them both in her deep blue cloak. The boys stopped trembling and felt once more safe and warm and snug.

The years passed, and one day the Christ Child was playing further away from home. He had gone to the forest with many other boys and girls. They were having a marvellous time, singing and laughing and skipping and dancing. Suddenly they heard a terrible howling. It came closer and closer and grew louder and louder. What was it, they wondered. A wolf? Or maybe a lion? They did not know, but they grew cold with fear. One of the children picked up a stick, another one climbed up into the nearest tree. Another child, shaking with fear, tried to hide behind a bush. But the Christ Child said: 'Come on, all of you, let's run as fast as we can to find Mother Mary. She will spread her deep blue mantle around us and then we won't have to fear anything in the whole wide world.'

'But how will Mother Mary's cloak be big enough for so many of us?' asked one of the girls.

'Don't worry about that,' said the Christ Child, 'Mother Mary's deep blue cloak can spread and spread and spread all over the world to hold every little child snug and cosy in its blueness.'

So the children ran out of the forest to find Mother Mary, and like the first night when the Christ Child was born, Mother Mary spread her blue cloak around all the boys and girls, keeping them warm, cosy and safe.

Mother Rabbit and the Bush Fire

This story is an example of the effect of an imaginative versus rational explanation for a four-year-old child who had been frightened by an experience of fire. See Chapter Three for the background to this story.

There was once a Mother Rabbit who lived in a hole in the ground in the middle of a green grassy field. This mother had many babies and every day the baby rabbits would enjoy playing, running and jumping in and out of the long grass around the edge of their home.

One day Mother Rabbit had to go away on a short journey. She left her babies sleeping, safe and snug in their rabbit hole, and set out across the field and along the dusty track. While she was away, a bushfire started up in a nearby gully, was given an extra push by the hot summer wind, and swept across the green grassy fields.

Later that day when Mother Rabbit was travelling back home, she saw to her horror that a fire had travelled before her. The green grassy field was now blackened stubble, and the ground was too hot for Mother Rabbit to walk on. 'Are my babies still safely asleep in their home?' she wondered.

Mother Rabbit had to wait till the cool of the evening before the ground was ready to step across. In the light of the twinkling stars, she made her way carefully to the edge of her rabbit hole, and peered down. What a relief to find that her babies were still sound asleep, safe and snug in their home. Mother Rabbit was so happy. She joined her babies down in the rabbit hole and they all slept till the next morning.

Every day the little rabbits watched their green grassy playground slowly grow back. It started first with little green shoots peeping out of the blackened ground. Taller and taller the little shoots grew, until the field was full of tall green grass once again. And once again, as before, the baby rabbits would enjoy playing, running and jumping in and out of the long grass around the edge of their home.

Born to be King

A story written for a six-year-old African boy (who was sexually abused at the age of three) to help heal his fear of going to the toilet. See Chapter One for more details of the background to this story.

There was once a child who was born to be King. When he was a little boy everyone called him the 'Little Prince', and he was given a golden crown to wear on his head.

Like all boys the Little Prince always liked exploring and climbing, running, jumping and having adventures. All day he would play in the gardens and forests of the palace with his friends. His crown sparkled in the sunlight and his friends loved to play close to its golden light.

However, it happened that one day, when he was playing with his friends near the palace wall, an older boy started to be rough in his playing. Suddenly he pushed the Little Prince so hard that he fell off the edge and landed far below on some rocks. Many bones in his body were broken – in both his legs and his arms.

The Little Prince was rescued by the palace workers and carried back to his bedroom deep inside the palace. There the doctors wrapped his arms and legs in strong bandages and for a long time he had to lie in his bed waiting for his bones to mend. In fact the Little Prince was in bed for so long that even when his bones were mended he had forgotten how to walk again. He just wanted to keep lying in his bed and no matter how much his father and mother pleaded with him to get up, he didn't even want to try to move.

One day his grandmother had an idea. She took her large hand mirror and went to the Little Prince's room and sat on his bed. Then she held the mirror up to him. 'You were born to be King' she said, 'and you have a golden crown on your head that likes to sparkle in the sunlight. But look at it now!'

The Little Prince looked in the mirror and was shocked to see that his golden crown, in the dark light of his bedroom, looked dull and grey. 'I must be carried outside,' he cried, 'so that my crown can sparkle in the sunlight once again.'

'No, you do not need to be carried,' replied his Grandmother, 'you must walk outside yourself ... but if you reach out your hand I will help you walk.'

The Little Prince reached out his hand and Grandmother helped him to slowly move his legs from the bed to the floor. Together they slowly walked out of the dark room, along the palace hallways and outside, into the garden and the sunshine.

It took many weeks before the Little Prince could run and jump and climb and have adventures as before, but every day all his friends came to hold his hands and help him walk. The more he moved around in the garden the more his golden crown would sparkle in the sunlight. Soon he was playing every day as before. His Grandmother would sit in a corner of the palace garden and watch him with his friends. She was so proud of her grandson, the Little Prince, who knew he was born to be King!

Follow up email from the boy's mother: 'My son is thrilled by his story, especially because he's a prince! (At my suggestion the mother had finger-knitted her son a crown from golden threads – see notes on the use of props in the section on Writing Therapeutic Stories.) He has been listening to it at bedtime, since that's the only time I have after my late night university class. He now goes to the toilet without my assistance. All I hear from time to time is the water flushing down the toilet. I am so excited to observe him overcome his phobia gradually. My worry about his toilet movements has soon passed. I hope and pray he'll have a smooth transition from daycare to school. The story has been of great help in my work, especially through experiencing the effect on the child of imaginative ideas that promote his emotional development.'

24

Illness, Grieving or Death

The Story of Silky Wriggly

A story for young children to explain terminal illness, or the death of a family member or close friend, in an imaginative way. Published by permission of the author, Susan Haris.

Once upon a time there was a village amongst the hills. In this village there was a white house. In the white house there lived a little girl who loved to look after silk worms. She kept them in a big open box, which she called Silk Worm Palace.

Very early every morning, when the sun came up from behind the hills, the little girl would run down to the creek where the Mulberry Tree grew.

'Dear Mulberry Tree, could I pick some of your shiny green leaves for my Silk Worms?'

'Of course,' the old Mulberry Tree would reply, 'I would be very happy to help your Silk Worms grow big and fat.'

Every day the little girl would thank the tree and pick some leaves and put them in her box. The tiny silk worms would gobble up the big leaves, one after another, and the worms grew bigger and bigger each day. They were wriggling and creeping and crawling around happily in their Palace, and growing bigger and fatter and fatter and bigger. The little girl laughed when she looked at them – she loved to watch them eat and grow and wriggle around day after day after day.

The little girl had one favourite silkworm. She called it Silky Wriggly. She would take it out of the box each day and let it crawl on her hands and arms, and talk to it and laugh with delight.

But one day when the little girl looked into the box she noticed that Silky Wriggly had stopped wriggling! 'What has happened?' the little girl wondered to herself, 'Has Silky Wriggly died?'

But the silk worm had not died, it had started to spin a very long golden thread to make a little golden cocoon. The other silk worms were also starting to do the same. All day long they spun and spun, and slowly all the silk worms changed into very quiet, golden cocoons, lying there very still in the bottom of the box.

The little girl was sad. She missed Silky Wriggly and all the other silkworms. It had been such fun to watch the lively silk worms creep and crawl, wriggle and grow. Now it was so very quiet.

One day the little girl was looking into the box and she said out loud: 'Silky Wriggly, I am missing you and your friends. It was so much fun watching you creep and crawl and wriggle and grow, but now it is very quiet and still. It makes me feel so sad.'

Just as she said this the golden cocoon that Silky Wriggly had spun around herself suddenly burst open and a moth flew out of it and landed on the edge of the box. The little girl could not believe her eyes. The moth's wings were so delicate and they glistened with many colours and patterns.

The moth flew around the little girl three times then settled on her hand and spoke to her in a clear voice. 'You know, I started to feel so uncomfortable in the cocoon. It was becoming too tight, I felt I was locked inside. But now that I've burst out of it I can leave it behind. Now I feel happy and free. I can fly up high in the sky, up to the golden sun. It is much more fun than the wriggling and creeping and crawling around that I used to enjoy when I was a silkworm. Goodbye little girl, and thank you for feeding me those delicious mulberry leaves. Now I don't need them anymore. Now I am free!'

And the beautiful moth flew out through the open window, high up in the sky, towards the golden sun.

Note: When telling stories such as this about death, the tale will gain in power if the teller really has a relationship to the idea that death is not the final end, but a radical transformation. Otherwise children, being extremely intuitive, may sense the doubt in the teller's mind and absorb this at the same time as the story.

Fly, Eagle, Fly

When I was working in South Africa in the late 1990s I listened to a radio interview with the Bishop of Table Bay (Cape Town). He described the following story that he told his eight-year-old daughter who was dying of cancer. It was taken from a folktale from Ghana with a 'resurrection theme', and the Bishop felt it had really helped the daughter and the whole family cope better with the reality of her coming death.

There was once an eagle chick that was born in a nest of chickens. A farmer had been walking in the mountains and had found the egg lying on the ground and had taken it home to his hen to help hatch it.

The eagle chick grew up with all the other chickens but always had a feeling it could fly high, but there was no one who could show it what to do ....

The farmer's boy took it and tried to help it – first from the top of a ladder, then from the roof of the house. But these two were not high enough for the eagle to really feel its wings.

Then the boy and the farmer took the eagle back to the mountains where it had come from and placed it on the edge of a high cliff. This time the eagle chick took off from the edge of the cliff and felt the air beneath its wings and the sun on its feathers and soared higher and higher.

Soon the eagle was back high up in the sky where it belonged and it flew up to the sun.

Stream, Desert, Wind

A beautiful story about change and transformation. This little tale is an anonymous gem re-written by the author. It could be used with age eight and older (and adults), accompanied by painting or drawing scenes from the stream's journey.

Like 'Fly Eagle Fly' and 'Silky Wriggly', this is another story of death and transformation. Something dies and is then reborn in a different way.

A stream was born high on a mountain. It rushed around stones, over waterfalls, across fields, and through forests and valleys. Finally it reached a great desert and pushed its water against the sand. Then the water disappeared. The stream, that was feeling so confident with its life up to this point, could not believe what was happening. 'My water is disappearing – how can I cross this desert?'

Then the stream heard a whispering. It seemed to be coming from the sand itself, 'Ask the wind – it knows a way to cross the desert.'

'The Wind can fly,' thought the stream. 'All I can do is disappear into the sand. I can't cross this desert.'

'Allow the wind to carry you,' the voice whispered. 'But then I will have to change. I don't want to change, I want to stay as I am.'

'If you continue to flow into the desert, you are changing – you are either going to disappear altogether or you will become a swamp.'

'But I want to stay myself,' said the stream. 'How can I get to the other side and still be myself?'

'If you remember your true self you will know this can never change,' whispered the voice.

The stream then remembered a long forgotten dream about being carried in the arms of the wind. It let go of the earth below and allowed itself to rise up in a vapour. The wind flew with it far across the desert, all the way to the mountains on the other side. Finally it was released as soft rain high on the top of a mountain.

With this the stream was born anew. It rushed around stones, over waterfalls, across fields, and through forests and valleys. And as it rushed along, it had watery memories of its true and essential self.

The Frog and the Pail of Cream

A Russian tale, retold by the author, to encourage strength and determination. Suitable for children and adults.

There was once a frog that jumped into a pail of cream. He swam round and round, kicking and splashing, trying to find a way out. Every so often he stopped to rest. He wondered if he would ever find a way out of his predicament.

Then he started to sing as he swam. He found the singing made him stronger.

I'm a little frog, and if I stay strong, I'll find a way out before too long!
The frog refused to give up.

He swam and swam, and sang and sang, until, without even realising it, his little feet had churned the cream into butter.

Finally he was able to climb up on the butter and hop out – just before the milkmaid came back for her pail!

The Little Clay Girl

A Tanzanian fairytale about death and transformation – re-written by the author. Suitable for age six and older.

There was once a man and his wife who lived together in a little house by a river on the edge of a forest. The man spent his days making wonderful things from the clay that he dug out of the banks of the river – pots and plates and cups and bowls. His wife worked all week growing vegetables in their garden – corn and cabbage and pumpkin and beans. On Saturdays they would load up their basket with the clay pieces and vegetables and carry them to market where they would sell their wares.

The couple were very happy with their life, except for one thing. They longed to have a child, but their house was empty of the laughter and dancing of little children.

One day the man was working with his clay, and singing as he worked:

Play and work, work and play, how I love to make things from clay!

The sun was shining brightly and the birds were singing as he worked, and he was feeling so happy that he had a most special thought:

I will make a little child from my clay today!

His clever hands set to work and in very little time he had made a beautiful little clay girl, with a shiny brown face and curly brown hair. When he was finished, he wrapped the little girl in a cloth dress, and lifted her up to carry her to the garden to show his wife. As he arrived at the garden where his wife was working, all of a sudden the little clay girl jumped down out of his hands and started to dance around.

His wife heard the lively noise and came running, and when she saw the little clay girl she bent down and hugged her dearly – 'At last we have a child to bring laughter and dancing into our home,' she cried.

From that day onwards the little clay girl lived with the man and his wife, and helped them with their work – sometimes with the man making clay pots and plates and cups and bowls, and sometimes with his wife in their garden, growing corn and cabbage and pumpkin and beans. The man and his wife were so happy to have a child in their home at last.

On Saturdays, when they travelled to market to sell their wares, they would leave the little clay girl at home to mind the house. They were worried that if it rained on the way, the rain would turn their new child back into a ball of clay.

'Stay close to the house, little clay girl,' they would say as they left for market, 'and if it starts to rain, make sure you wait inside for us until we return.'

The little clay girl always did as they said, and each week the man and his wife would return from market to find her waiting safely inside the house for them.

One Saturday however, while the clay girl was home by herself, she heard the laughter and dancing of a group of children as they passed by the house. The children were on their way to the forest to pick fresh berries, and the little clay girl couldn't help but follow their laughter and song. All the way to the forest she went, and joined in with the dancing and berry picking. When the children's baskets were full to overflowing with ripe juicy berries, they set out to return home, with the little clay girl dancing along beside them. But just before she reached her house, some storm clouds passed overhead and the rain poured down from the sky as if God himself was tipping buckets from the clouds.

When the man and his wife returned from market, the house was empty and they couldn't find the little clay girl anywhere. The rain had stopped but there were puddles everywhere up and down the road. They looked towards the forest, and there they saw a ball of clay lying in the grass at the edge of the trees. Straight away they knew what had happened to their little clay child!

The man carefully picked up the ball of clay and carried it home to his workshop and put it in his most special clay pot.

His wife placed the pot by their front door, and everyday they would water a few drops into the pot and remember the little girl that they missed so much.

Then one day they noticed a little green shoot pushing up out of the clay, and day by day they watched it grow. It grew and grew, sprouting little leaves and then a rich red bud, and one day it blossomed into a most beautiful red rose.

From this time onwards, the rose bush continued to flower with a new rose every day, and the man went back to making pots and plates and cups and bowls, and singing as he worked:

Play and work, work and play, how I love to make things from clay!

And the wife went back to growing corn and cabbage and pumpkin and beans, and singing as she dug in the garden:

Play and work, work and play, how I love to make things from clay!

And from this time on, every Saturday they would load up their basket with the clay pieces and the vegetables and a bunch of beautiful fresh roses, and carry it to market where they would sell their wares.

A Doll for Sylvia

Sylvia was orphaned at the age of five after her whole family was killed in a raid on her village – she has now been adopted by the SOS Children's Village in Nairobi where she will live until the age of eighteen. Sylvia's story was told to her by her class teacher and was followed up with Sylvia finding a special doll, dressed in clothes embroidered with silver and gold threads, waiting in her bed the next morning. In her new house, the family 'mother' noticed a great change in her play and general interaction with others after this story. See Chapter Five for more background to this story.

Sylvia's mother and father were safe in heaven. All their children were with them except for little Sylvia who had stayed behind on earth.

At night in the light of the twinkling stars they could see their little daughter asleep in her bed. They were so happy that she had a safe new home and a new mother to take care of her. But they could see that their daughter was sad and lonely sometimes and they wanted to send down a gift from heaven – the gift of a little friend for Sylvia to play with and to sleep with at night.

With the help of heaven's angels they gathered golden threads from the sun and silver threads from the moon, and on the heavenly weaving loom they wove a special cloth to use to make a little doll.

When the doll was ready one of heaven's angels cradled it in her arms and travelled with it across the sky of twinkling stars and down to earth. When she arrived at Sylvia's new house she reached in through the window and tucked the doll into the bed next to Sylvia's sleeping head.

The next morning when Sylvia woke up her new gift was waiting to greet her. The doll's dress sparkled gold and silver in the morning light and Sylvia was so happy to see her. She knew it was a heavenly gift . She named it … and the doll became her special friend.

Shimmer Wing By Sandra Frain

Shimmer Wing is a story that was written to tell at the ceremony of a young girl, Shalem, who had passed away a few months before her fourth birthday after being bitten by a snake.

For more background on the writing of this story, see Chapter 32, page 274.

First the setting (as described by Sandra): We gathered, at 4 p.m. on Sunday 18 February 2007, on the sandy edge of a wide tidal creek where Shalem loved to play and swim.

As the tide moved out, at the first point of sand in the middle of the creek that showed itself above the water line, a wooden totem pole was carried out and ceremoniously raised. The totem pole had been made by Shalem's father, mother, and family friends. The totem pole was carved with angel wings at its three-quarter mark, with an owl, some dolphins, a whale, a turtle and a serpent exquisitely adorning its length. In the centre was a picture of Shalem set in a carved heart.

Near the base was an altar upon which there was a vessel containing Shalem's ashes. People placed gifts to Shalem there. All around the totem, in the sand, curved a spiral where people placed colourful blossoms and stones and shells. A fire was lit in a brazier, burning sacred herbs and resins.

Children played in the sand, mounding and dripping the wet sand into castles. The family thanked people for coming to celebrate Shalem's wonderful life. I was introduced as her daycare teacher and proceeded to tell my story.

After the story, people shared memories of Shalem, sang songs and played music inspired by and dedicated to Shalem. People placed individual prayer ties in the fire. Shalem's parents offered Shalem's ashes to the incoming tidal water of the Pacific Ocean. The totem was carried like a cross out of the creek. The colourful blossoms and stones on the spiral tossed about as the tide filled up the creek. Votive candles floated out to sea.

Families were given a birdwing vine to take home to plant in their own gardens (in the story, the yellow bellflower from the 'birdwing' vine is Shimmer Wing's best friend).

Once upon a time in a very wet rainforest there lived so many friends that you could never count them all. These friends talked to each other and played with each other and they worked together and they even fought sometimes like good friends do!

One of these friends was a brilliant blue butterfly called 'Shimmer Wing'. Shimmer Wing' butterfly loved to play 'peek-a-boo'. You would see her flying about as blue as blue could be and then, whit, she was gone. But if you looked carefully you would see that she had hidden the blue side of her wings and now she looked like a brown leaf on a tree branch. Very tricky she was. This was her song:

> *I'm flash of blue. How do you do?*
> *Can you see me? Peek-a–boo. I see you!*
> (Sandra waved a blue scarf through the
> air and then hid it behind her)

Shimmer Wing's best friend was Yellow Bell-Flower. Shimmer Wing knew that she was in for a tasty treat of Yellow Bell's nectar when she saw her yellow flower. She tickled Yellow Bell with her butterfly tootsies when she landed on Yellow Bell's petals. Yum yum mmm, she sipped Yellow Bell's nectar with her long butterfly tongue (and the teeny butterfly eggs inside her grew a little bit bigger).

In the wet rainforest Yellow Bell lived next to a bush. Under this bush lived Satin Bower Bird. In Satin Bower Bird's nest lay many blue things – a blue pin, a piece of blue string, a shiny blue lolly wrap and even some of his own blue feathers. Having lots of blue things in his home was a good way to make friends! Shimmer Wing liked to tease him by flying past his bower and dazzling him with her own brilliant blue wings as she looked at his collection.

What a perfect place to lay her butterfly eggs above Satin Bower Bird's blue treasures! Lots of leaves for her greedy larvae babies to eat when they hatched! So close to her best friend Yellow Bell (whom her babies could visit when they grew their wings).

One night Shimmer Wing saw a light in the sky that was different to her friends the stars. This light was like a starry ball with a magnificent tail behind it. It had an even bigger tail than that noisy Lyre-Bird neighbour who always made such a racket mimicking this bird and that animal.

Shimmer Wing flew up to Grandpa Koala who was sitting in a top branch of Grandfather Gum Tree. 'What is that light up there in the sky, Grandfather Koala?'

Grandpa Koala chewed on his gum leaves and didn't answer

for a while. He shifted his big bottom on the Grandfather Gum Tree branch where he was sitting and he cleared his throat as grandfathers do.

'It is like a giant broom sweeping the heavens and collecting good things. It showers presents onto Mother Earth too,' he said.

'What kind of presents?' asked Shimmer Wing.

Grandfather Koala answered, 'Presents like colours, and brightness, and goodness.' Grandfather Koala cleared his throat again – 'We eat the presents and we climb them and we breathe them and we walk on them. And', he added, 'it collects presents from Mother Earth too.'

'Oh,' said Shimmer Wing. Then she flew down and laid her eggs underneath a big leaf inside the leafy bush of Satin Bower Bird's bower. When she finished she heard a 'neighghgh'. It was her friend, Frangipani Unicorn.

'Frangipani Unicorn, will you take me up to visit the light?' Shimmer Wing fluttered by Frangipani's tall white ear. Frangipani Unicorn could leap over rainbows when she wanted to. Frangipani was kind and she was gentle and she was very strong.

Frangipani Unicorn closed her eyes and imagined herself leaping up, up, up, into the sky to the bright light.

'I can try,' she neighed softly. Frangipani Unicorn trotted and cantered and galloped so fast that she rose up in to the sky with Shimmer Wing hiding inside her tall white ear. Up, up, up, they flew to where fluff and puff clouds played peek-a-boo with the bright light of the comet's magnificent tail.

'I love you,' Shimmer Wing fluttered, waving her wings to Frangipani Unicorn. Frangipani Unicorn galloped back through the cloudy and starry sky to her home on Mother Earth.

In the morning the forest was calm. The Bangalow Palms were waving their fronds graciously. The dew fairies sparkled on the rocks and trees. The light of the Mighty Sun and the pitter-patter raindrop fairies made colourful rainbows everywhere. Frangipani Unicorn was practising jumping over them and under them and even through them all.

Grandpa Koala felt wiser as he sat in his Gum Tree chewing on his gum leaves and pondering on the brightness of the comet and its magnificent tail of light.

Satin Bower Bird found pretty blue angel wings in front of his bower! Yellow Bell's petals shimmered and smelt more beautiful than ever.

All of Shimmer Wing's friends were brighter and more beautiful than ever before. All of Shimmer Wing's friends were filled with her 'shimmer' for ever and ever.

25

New Baby in the House

The Magic Stick

A story for a five-year-old girl who was soon to have a new baby brother. Her parents were concerned that their first and only daughter might be jealous of the new baby and not accept him. The story helped greatly to motivate her acceptance and involvement. It was strengthened by the mother helping her daughter make a magic stick with coloured pieces of wool, feathers and shells.

There was once a little girl who was feeling bored with her play and toys. She was sitting under a spreading tree at the bottom of her garden, when all of a sudden a small stick broke off the tree and fell to the ground. It landed right next to her, and strangely enough it started to sing to her:

> *Wrap me up in colours bright; keep me safe both day and night –*
> *And when there's magic in the air, I'll lead you to a treasure fair!*

The girl was very excited to hear the stick singing. 'This must be a magic stick,' she thought, and she picked it up and carried it home. When she reached her house she went straight to the basket in the lounge room where her mother kept balls of coloured wool. One by one she started to wrap the stick in bright colours. Then she took it to her room and found a safe place for it to live on the table next to her bed.

When she woke the next morning she could hear the magic stick singing to her.

Today there's magic in the air – I'll lead you to a treasure fair!

Picking up the stick, she felt it start to shake and it seemed to say 'Follow me'. She let the stick show her where to go and it led her out into the garden, right down to where some beautiful birds' feathers had been left on the grass. 'This must be the treasure fair,' thought the little girl, and she decided to tie the feathers to her magic stick to make it more beautiful than before.

The next morning when she woke up the magic stick was singing to her again.

Today there's magic in the air – I'll lead you to a treasure fair!
She followed the magic stick out of her house and across to the beach, and there on the golden sands lay some pretty shells, all pink and white and patterned bright. 'This must be the treasure fair,' thought the little girl, and she decided to tie the shells to her magic stick to make it more beautiful than before.

The next morning when she woke up the magic stick was singing to her again.

Today there's magic in the air – I'll lead you to a treasure fair!

But this time the magic stick did not lead her out of the house. Instead it sang all the way up the hall and into her mother's and father's room. There on the bed were her parents with a tiny new baby lying between them. The baby was wrapped up in a warm blanket. 'This is indeed a treasure fair,' thought the little girl, and she held her magic stick with its bright colours and beautiful feathers and shells up for the little baby to see. The baby smiled and the little girl felt so happy inside that she thought she would burst!

From that day to this, the magic stick has helped this little girl have many adventures and find many treasures. But her most favourite 'treasure fair' was finding a new baby all wrapped up in a warm blanket on her parents' bed.

The Water Child

A story for a four-year-old boy to help introduce the news of a baby sister joining the family. The watery theme was chosen to link with the water birth that the mother had planned to have at home.

Once upon a time there was a little boy who had a very special friend. This friend was not like all his other friends. This friend lived far away, up in Cloud Heaven, high in the sky.

The little boy could sometimes hear his friend whispering down to him when he was out in the garden. And sometimes in his dreams at night the boy would visit Cloud Heaven and the two children would play happily together, rolling and tumbling in the soft whiteness, and jumping from cloud to cloud.

One day his special friend decided it was time to leave her cloud home and come down and live on the earth with the little boy's family.

The special friend said goodbye to everyone in Cloud Heaven. Then the Lady of the Rain wrapped her in a violet cloak and carried her down with her next shower of raindrops. She placed her softly into the world below, in a big pool of cooling water.

The boy's mother and father were waiting for her. They lifted her up and out of the water pool and showed her to the little boy. 'This is your new baby sister' they said, 'and she is called Laila.' She has come to live with us. She needs a little time to grow and get used to being in the world, but soon she will be ready to play with you.'

It was a most beautiful day and the boy's family was so happy to have a new child come to live in their home. The little boy made some pictures for the walls of the baby's room and collected brightly coloured leaves and flowers for a mobile to hang over the baby's bed. Sometimes he would hold his new little sister in his arms and hug her and sing lullabies to her.

Soon Laila had grown big enough to crawl around, and then walk and then run.

In no time at all it was Laila's first birthday and the little boy was helping her open her first birthday present.

It was a beautiful golden ball!

The little boy rolled it across the floor and his sister rolled it back to him. The little boy laughed and his sister laughed too. Together they played with the golden ball, laughing and having such fun, just as they had once played together in heaven.

26

Separation Anxiety

The Monkey Tree

'The Monkey Tree' was written by a family daycare worker, Jilly Norris, for a four-year-old girl whose parents had separated. The child was finding it difficult adapting to the new shared-custody arrangements. She had 3 teenage siblings and her home life was often noisy and a little 'chaotic' (which is why Jilly chose the monkey theme). This story could be adapted to suit a variety of ages and predicaments relating to separation and separation anxiety. (See Chapter 32 for a more detailed account of the effect of this story).

Once upon a time, in the middle of a jungle, there was a family of cheeky monkeys who all lived together in their monkey tree.

> *They were as busy, cheeky and noisy as could be,*
> *They chattered and laughed in their monkey tree,*
> *They swung from their tails and scratched their fleas,*
> *and played together happily.*

One small monkey whose name was Mali was learning from her big brothers and sisters how to make a night-time nest in the monkey tree, by bending and tucking the soft branches and leaves together to make a cosy bed. It was not easy and sometimes Mali would fall through the bottom of the nest. But after much practice she learned to make her bed properly, so that she could sleep in it as cosy as cosy can be.

Mali slept in her night-time nest as cosy as can be,
Surrounded by the nests of her monkey family.

One morning Mali was playing with her cousins when there was a rumbling sound in the sky. Mali took no notice, but her older brothers and sisters and cousins began to chatter more loudly than ever and climbed to the top of the monkey tree to see what they could see.

Dark rain clouds began to gather in the sky, the thunder rumbled and lightning crashed. Rain began to fall and the wind began to blow. The monkeys all huddled together in the middle of the tree to wait for the storm to pass. They were very quiet… Suddenly there was a loud cracking and creaking noise and a big branch broke away from their monkey tree and tumbled down to the ground far below.

Eventually, the rain stopped falling and the wind stopped blowing and the dark clouds moved away so that the monkeys could see and feel the warm sun again.

Because one big branch was gone from their tree, some of the monkeys had to go and make their night-time nests in a neighbouring tree. So now the monkeys were very busy.

Mali thought it was rather exciting to go and visit some of her family in another tree and she made a nest there too, just in case she decided to sleep over.

Now the family of monkeys lived in two monkey trees, and once again…

They were as busy, cheeky and noisy as could be,
They chattered and laughed in their monkey trees,
They swung from their tails and scratched their fleas,
and played together happily.

And Mali now had nests in two monkey trees, so that…

Mali slept in her night-time nests as cosy as can be,
Surrounded by the nests of her monkey family.

Mother Moon

This story was written for a five-year-old whose mother suddenly left home, leaving the boy with relatives (the mother returned 5 months later). The story not only helped the child feel stronger, but it helped his relatives too. It is included here by permission of the author, Alison Brooking.

Once upon a time there was a Child Star who was happy playing in the sky with the other stars. He was always shining, and in the night time when his Mother the Moon was there, all the children on earth could see him even when it was dark. In the daytime he was still shining but no one could see him because Father Sun was so big and bright that he outshone all the stars.

As Father Sun went to sleep, the Moon would rise and come and remind her star children to shine brightly on the earth all through the night, to help the children there. She would polish them and look after them, and together they would shine silver beams down onto earth, so that all the little night animals could see their food and so that all the plants could grow. The Child Star liked to be near Mother Moon and he could feel her soft moonbeams touching him too.

One evening, as the last of the sun's rays were shining on the earth, Child Star was waiting for Mother Moon to come along on her nightly visit to all the stars. He waited a long time with his friends in the sky, but she did not come. All the stars waited and it became very dark and cold, and Child Star began to feel sad. Then he thought to himself – it will be very dark down on the earth for the possums and owls and children, if Mother Moon isn't shining down her moonbeams. He decided that Mother Moon would like it if he polished himself and made himself so bright that it wouldn't be so dark on earth. So he was very brave and he rubbed and polished himself until he was shining so brightly, and then he told his brother and sister star children to do the same.

Down on the earth, a little girl was sitting looking out of her bedroom window into the dark, dark night, waiting for the moon to rise. She felt cold, sitting there for so long, but she wanted to see the stars twinkling and feel the moonbeams on her face. This was her favourite part of the evening – after her mother had sung her a goodnight song she would tiptoe out of bed and sit at her window looking up at the sky. But on this evening she started to yawn and yawn and rub her eyes because it was pitch dark around her. Just as she was nodding off to sleep she saw one little star begin to twinkle all on its own. The star grew brighter and brighter and it felt as though it was shining down just on her. It was Child Star! Then another star and another started to shine, until at last the sky was filled with bright twinkling stars that seemed to be so happy, even as if they were talking to each other. This made the little girl so happy and at last she went to sleep.

The next morning, when Father Sun spread his warm sunbeams out across the sea and the hills, Child Star was fast asleep, tired after his long night's work. He had never had to shine so brightly on his own before. He dreamt that his dear Mother Moon was talking to him and she was saying 'I am very proud of what a wonderful brave and shining star you have become, Child Star. Soon I will come back and shine in the sky again, but until then you will have to play with your friends and polish each other at night, so you can still shine light down onto the earth. To help you with the shining, you can catch some of Father Sun's warm sunbeams as he goes down at the end of the day, and if you are very careful with them, he will help you to use them properly. I love you, Child Star, and I think of you all the time. Goodnight, Child Star.'

That night Child Star awoke and heard his mother's words inside him and he knew that he wasn't alone and he didn't have to feel so sad. He remembered what she said. The next evening, instead of trying to shine so brightly all by himself, he asked Father Sun if he could catch some of his last golden rays to store up, and in this way he became the brightest star in the sky.

Baby Bear Koala

A therapeutic story for 'separation anxiety', written for a four-year-old boy who was having difficulty parting from his mother at pre-school. See Chapter Four for the unpredictable consequence of this story.

Mother Bear Koala and her baby lived high up in the tallest gum tree in the forest. All day long Mother Bear climbed from branch to branch, picking juicy gum leaves to feed her hungry baby. When all the best leaves on one branch were finished, up to the next branch she would go, with Baby Bear Koala holding tightly onto her back.

> *Mother Bear Koala sitting in a tree*
> *Baby Bear Koala crying 'I'm hun-gry'!*
> *Picking juicy leaves for breakfast and for lunch,*
> *Eating juicy leaves, munchety-crunch.*
> *Picking juicy leaves for lunch and for tea,*
> *Eating juicy leaves, munchety-dee.*

When all the best leaves on this branch were finished, down to another branch Mother Bear would go, with her baby holding tightly onto her back.

> *Mother Bear Koala sitting in a tree*
> *Baby Bear Koala crying 'I'm hun-gry'!*
> *Picking juicy leaves for breakfast and for lunch,*
> *Eating juicy leaves, munchety-crunch.*
> *Picking juicy leaves for lunch and for tea,*
> *Eating juicy leaves, munchety-dee.*

There were so many branches on the gum tree. Every day Mother Bear Koala would move to a new branch to find fresh juicy gum leaves for her baby. Every day, up or down she would climb, with Baby Bear Koala on her back. He was always so hungry!

And every day Baby Bear Koala was growing bigger and bigger, eating juicy gum leaves for breakfast, lunch and tea – and growing bigger and bigger and bigger! As he grew bigger and bigger he grew heavier and heavier, until he was so heavy that it was difficult for Mother Bear to lift him onto her back – and even more difficult for her to climb up and down the tree with him.

Mother Bear Koala was growing very tired from all this hard work. Then one day, while she was sitting in the fork of the tree and Baby Bear Koala was crying – I'm hun-gry! – Mother Bear Koala was so, so tired that she fell asleep right there! And she was so fast asleep that Baby Bear could not wake her, no matter how loud he cried.

Eventually Baby Bear Koala climbed off his mother's back and sat on the branch next to his sleeping mother. Up above him he could see some yummy leaves to eat – he was so hungry! How he would love to pick those juicy leaves for his lunch. How he would love to eat those juicy leaves, munchety-crunch!

Then Baby Bear Koala thought – maybe I am big enough to climb up and pick those juicy leaves by myself. He sat for a while – those leaves looked so juicy.

Then he started to climb up the trunk – he was a little bit scared but it was easier to do than he thought. His baby claws had grown long and sharp and strong. They dug into the tree trunk and stopped him from sliding down.

Up and up he went, higher and higher, until finally he reached the next branch. He crawled along a little way, slowly and carefully. Looking down he could see his mother asleep in the fork of the tree below. He was so high and he felt so brave. Right in front of him were some juicy leaves, so he picked some for his lunch, and he sat high up in the tree all by himself, eating juicy leaves, munchety-crunch.

Later that day Mother Koala Bear woke up and looked around. Where was her baby? She looked down – had he fallen off her back and out of the tree? Baby Bear Koala was nowhere to be seen! Then she heard a munchety-crunch noise and looked up. There was her baby, on a higher branch – not a baby anymore, but a little koala bear, all by himself, having his lunch.

Mother Koala Bear smiled a very big smile. Then she climbed up the tree and sat next to little koala bear. Together they picked juicy leaves for lunch and for tea, and together they ate juicy leaves, munchety-dee.

SECTION FIVE

THE ART OF STORYTELLING

Stories need to be told to really come alive! So far the emphasis in this book has been on story content – with little mention of story delivery.

In this section some attention will be given to storytelling techniques and a variety of presentation ideas. Please accept this as a 'taster' only, not a comprehensive guide. The subject of storytelling, one of the oldest known art forms, is very extensive and culturally rich. The Storytelling unit that I developed for Southern Cross University is a course lasting 150 hours, and even this is not long enough to fully explore the topic.

Two books that provide excellent and detailed guidance for the keen storyteller are *Storytelling and the Art of Imagination* and *Storytelling with Children,* both by Nancy Mellon. These and many other references, including storytelling websites are listed at the back of the book.

27

Storytelling and Story Reading

Telling stories

What is the difference between telling or reading a story? I was once working in a holiday daycare centre, and taking the most of the opportunity to include a storytelling session every day of the week. One seven-year-old boy, who was obviously enjoying the experience, said to me, 'You know Susan, I think 'person' stories are much better than 'book' stories.'

I have also been asked, 'Do you come from a different land?' by a child in my audience who had just heard stories 'told' for the first time in his life. Children notice the difference between telling and reading, even if they are not old enough to articulate or fully understand what it is. Storytelling is very different to story reading. In storytelling the sharing of the story is more personal – the storyteller connects more directly with the audience through eyes, gesture, voice and proximity. Not bound by the words in the book, the teller is also free to use his own words within the framework of the story. This freedom of language and movement add to the personal nature of storytelling.

Storytelling allows much more room for the child's imagination. Rather than the pictures in a picture book providing the images, the storyteller's words stimulate the listener to create mental pictures of the story. The storyteller's face, voice, body and personality also help to convey mood and meaning. One of the most common remarks from my storytelling classes is that the best thing about listening to a 'told' story is that there is no book getting in the way of the story experience.

Maureen Watson, an indigenous Australian storyteller, says told stories 'touch' the audience. I have experienced this many times – through eyes, voice and gestures the storyteller spins out invisible threads from her body that 'touch' the listeners, and can thus 'hold' them in her grasp from start to finish. In fact, this is often a way for the storyteller to quieten a restless child. With a quick flash of eye contact, or a change in voice or hand gesture, the child receives a direct message without the storyteller needing to move from her place or deviate from the story. Usually 'homeopathic' messages are suitable for the little ones, increasing to stronger doses for older children!

The 'holding' power of storytelling can help develop and strengthen concentration. This ability is much lacking in many 'TV' children today, who are used to sitting passively in front of a screen and being entertained. During a one-year storytelling programme in my kindergarten I have many times observed remarkable changes in the children's concentration. Five-year-old children who can hardly sit still for two minutes in Term One, can concentrate deeply for at least fifteen to twenty minutes at story time by the end of the year. This concentration is carried into other activities, and is one of the most important preparations and skills necessary for formal learning.

For the above educational reasons, storytelling is very valuable at school. For the pre-school and kindergarten ages, repetition of the same story is an important part of the programme for young children (as discussed in previous chapters, they thrive on the repetition); for primary ages, as the stories grow in length, the teacher can experiment with telling a part of a story each day, having the children recount it the following day, then continuing on with the next section or chapter of the story. This exercise also strengthens concentration and memory

Reading stories

Although the 'told' experience is undoubtedly a more lively and personal way of sharing a story, both telling and reading are important ways of delivering or presenting stories. There is a place for both in our role as carers of young children. Especially with the dominance of 'screen' media in children's lives today, having stories told and/or read by adults is a wonderful blessing. Sometimes, especially in one-to-one situations, the 'book' can be a bridge that brings a closeness through sitting side by side, or, for a young child, on the adult's lap.

During story reading with picture books, the child or children use the illustrations to help understand and appreciate the story. There is often occasional eye contact between reader and listeners, and this helps to build the connection between them. If the reader knows the story quite well, he can improvise with the wording in some places and use the sequence of pictures like a 'prop' for storytelling. If reading the exact words, then the reader should experiment with ways to make sure the audience has a clear view of the pictures, either holding the picture up at the end of each page of words, or holding the book permanently within view so the pictures are accessible to all the children in the audience. For a teacher, it helps to be well prepared by reading the story beforehand.

There are many beautiful picture books on the market that are a delight for both adult and child to share. For help in choosing these, the age-appropriate indications given earlier in this book apply. A golden rule is to avoid anything that has strong or scary images for the younger ones. This follows the same logic as the importance of 'happy and hope-filled endings' to feed the growing child.

For older children, who have outgrown most picture books, and who can usually read by themselves, it is wonderful for teachers and parents to still continue a ritual of shared reading, from both classic poetry collections and favourite novels. These experiences will be remembered for a lifetime. I still enjoy being read to by my husband sometimes, before falling into a deep and very relaxed sleep.

> Storytelling is born out of the oral tradition.
> Story reading depends on the written text.
> Both are important ways of sharing stories

Most important is for you to have your own experience of the difference between telling and reading. If there is a storytelling group, or a teacher/storyteller near you, go along to the local school or library and listen. Or experiment with your friends – see if they will read to you and then tell a story to you. They could even use the daily news or 'gossip' as their stories – both read and told. After all, we tell stories in an informal way to each other all the time.

Storytelling techniques and rituals

The best way to become a storyteller is to tell stories! Through the practice of storytelling you will learn surprising lessons. The art of storytelling is personal and individual. Every storyteller and every audience is different. Every time a story is told it is a new and different experience.

However, despite the personal nature of the art of storytelling, there are some helpful tips and techniques worth reading about and trying out. I have tried to summarise these in the following pages.

Storytelling – a 'sharing'

The best advice I can offer to you when starting to tell stories is to continually remind yourself that the experience of storytelling is 'sharing' rather than 'performance'. This sense can minimise the tension you may feel about sharing a story for the first time ... the experience should be enjoyable for both you and your listeners. In fact they will enjoy it most if you do!

Another tip is to imagine yourself as part of the 'world-wide-story-web', keeping alive the special stories that you find through telling them to others. This imaginative vision can help remind you that you are not alone in your telling, but one of millions of people around the world who are sharing stories with each other.

Being well-prepared will also help you feel relaxed. Unless you have the rare quality of being a natural storyteller, this preparation may be hard work and laborious. But once you really 'know' a story well, it lives in your resource kit forever.

Preparation for telling

There are different ways of preparing and learning stories:
- Memorising word by word
- Memorising through sequencing or framing the images – i.e. visualising in your imagination the scenes in the story journey in correct sequence. If it helps, you can summarise or sketch these on paper.
- Improvising – having a basic sequence, possibly with the story beginning and ending well rehearsed, then improvising the rest.

Whichever way you find easiest, it is important to actually use your voice in your practise sessions, and not just 'think' the story through. The process of bringing the story 'down' (from your head into your voice) is an important one for a storyteller's preparation.

Creating story rituals

Creating simple rituals for storytelling helps to build the mood and encourage the audience to listen from the first moment. A story ritual helps the teller and the audience to cross the bridge from the busy everyday world into the realm of story. This can be as simple as the storyteller playing some music before the story. In many cultures the main ritual or tradition for stories was that they were told at night around the fire, creating a connection between time and place.

In the home environment, the ritual may be as simple as lighting a candle at bedtime and singing a lullaby at the end of the story. Or telling a short story or funny story at the end of the evening meal. Or establishing a tradition of shared storytelling on long walks or car journeys.

In the professional environment, a therapist or counsellor could have a story bag or box (with props and puppets inside), or a sand tray with animals and figurines. Stories could arise from these each time the child comes to visit.

In my teaching work my rituals have varied depending on my venue and audience, but have been known to include any or all of the following:

- Playing music (before and after the story)
- Lighting a candle or lantern
- Sitting on a special 'story' chair or stool
- Arranging a story corner or table for props and puppets
- Having a set time in the rhythm of the day for 'story'
- Helping bring children into a 'listening mood' by using some finger games before the story
- Leading the children into the room with a 'story' song

Example of a story song
(used in East Africa to lead the kindergarten children inside for story time – in English and Kiswahili)

Come with me to a fairytale land
To a land where stories unfold,
Follow the rainbow over the bridge
Into the garden of gold.

Fungua mlango kwa hadithi za kale
Hapo mahala kwenye shamba la hadithi
Fuata mwenge kwenye shamba la dhahabu.

For older primary children the situation is usually more direct and less ritualistic. The teacher/storyteller often needs to stand, not sit, in front of the class to tell the story.

When telling stories to older children, a standing position may be necessary to allow a more dramatic telling style – the age group and the contents of the myths, legends and other story genres will probably demand this. However, there will also be times when, to soothe or quieten an excited class, or to suit the mood of the particular story, the teacher may choose to sit and tell it, adopting the simpler, less dramatic storytelling style that is most suited to younger children (see also Chapter 31).

No matter what age the audience, though, playing an instrument (guitar, small harp, drum) works well to mark the beginning of the story and 'bring in' the listeners.

At fairs and festivals I have danced through a crowd playing a recorder like a Pied Piper to gather up the audience. I once set up a storytelling tipi with a magic stepping stone pathway leading to the entrance – this proved to be a wonderful house for storytelling. I have also sat under a tree blowing enormous bubbles to attract the attention of the children, then started my session with a bubble story.

28

Multi-Cultural Thoughts

Cultural sensitivity

Being sensitive to other cultures is something one needs to consider when telling and writing stories. I first learnt about this when working with Xhosa teachers in Cape Town. I was suggesting ideas for a healing story that included a monkey. The group went quiet then a teacher spoke up. 'It is considered bad luck to have a monkey in a story,' she said. She didn't want to elaborate, so I didn't push for an explanation. The monkey was taken out of the story and, after checking for suggestions and approval, a rabbit leapt into its place!

This experience taught me to do more thorough research when working in other countries and with other cultures. Sometimes this can be as simple as having a chat with one of my indigenous colleagues at breaktime, or going online or to a library. For a teacher of a multi-cultural group, a child's parents would be a good first source of information.

The healing nature of multi-cultural tales

Folk- and fairytales contain something of the unique quality of the culture from which they are drawn. By telling folktales from diverse cultures we can help to strengthen our children's global rather than just national consciousness. An American Indian storyteller once told me she believed the 'timbre' of a people's stories conveyed their heart qualities.

Any classroom dedicated to promoting multiculturalism should have an abundance of folktales available. Such stories are a healing balm for our modern times. As well as enriching all children, experience has shown that minority children, in particular, 'light up' when they hear a story drawn from their own culture. This acknowledgement of a child's cultural background can be both reassuring and strengthening.

When telling indigenous stories, it is respectful to research the history and meaning behind the tales (see website references at back of book). Before telling such stories, it is also respectful to question how appropriate it is for a non-indigenous person to do this. I have found most cultural communities quite open and enthusiastic here – our common interest in storytelling seems to build bridges. Also, asking permission to tell a story is very different from requesting to print it.

In Groome's book on *Teaching Aboriginal Studies Effectively*, the chapter on 'Stories of the Dreaming' is a help to storytellers who wish to share stories from indigenous Australian culture. Groome suggests that any teller of the Dreaming Stories needs to understand the history and the range of purposes of such stories – from teaching spiritual realities to teaching behaviour and values. They are stories of 'beginnings', and, according to Maureen Watson, a well-known indigenous Australian storyteller, they are just as relevant today as they were in the past. Although I have respectfully told Aboriginal Dreamtime stories, I have not included any in print form in this book. Their ownership lies with groups of indigenous elders, not just one person, and it is considered inappropriate for a non-indigenous person to seek permission for their written use.

Different story rituals for different cultures

As you investigate ways of storytelling in different cultures, you will find many different rituals for starting and finishing stories. There are many more ways to begin a story than *Once upon a time ...*

Story beginnings
* *On a day like today, in a place not far away ...*
* *A story, a story, let it come, let it go! ...* (West African)
* Storyteller: *Hadithi Hadithi – A story, a story;* audience: *Hadithi njoo! – Story come!* (East African)
* *Yool-burroo boura – these things happened a long time ago .....* (Indigenous Australian – used with some Dreamtime Stories)

- *Mother has a treasure, a treasure for her children – what do you think the treasure is? The treasure is a story! ...* (South African)
- *Once there was, and once there was not ...*
- *Once upon a time, it could have happened here, it could have happened there, it could have happened anywhere ...*

Story endings

- *A story, a story, let it come, let it go! ...* (West African)
- *Hadithi Hadithi, Maziwa ya watoto wote! – A story, a story, milk for all the children! –* (East African)
- *Mother had a treasure, a treasure for her children – what do you think the treasure was? The treasure was a story! ...* (South African)
- *Phela, phela ntsomi* – traditional Xhosa ritual meaning 'end of story'
- *And now you can have your supper, say your prayers and go to bed ... Morning is wiser than evening.* (Russian)

I encourage you to experiment with some of the above, or even make up your own. This particularly applies to any that relate to your own culture, and/or the culture of the story you are telling and of the children in your class or audience (after checking with the parents of a child from the relevant culture, of course). However, be careful and sensitive – some of these ideas may not suit who you are, your personal background, and where you live. They may just not feel right to you.

29

Storytelling for Different Audiences and Occasions

Polarities in storytelling

In planning your storytelling for different audiences and occasions, it helps to be aware of the many different kinds of stories there are. Most stories occupy a position somewhere on several of the following continuums:

- short to long
- funny to serious
- local to global/universal
- simple to complex
- general to specific
- real to imaginary

The list could go on – stories that are strong and dramatic to stories that are light and frivolous; stories with or without audience participation; stories that are full of rhyme and/or song ...

The environmental fairytale, 'Garden of Light' (see page 127), is imaginary, medium to long, serious, quite complex and with universal relevance. 'The Antelope, The Butterfly and The Chameleon' (see page 224) is a folktale that is imaginary but with real elements. It is also funny, but with a serious lesson to be learnt about facing fears.

If you are getting confused, don't be alarmed. It is probably because the very nature of stories doesn't allow them to be neatly boxed and sorted. However, one good reason to be aware of the possible continuums is to help you plan an appropriate mix in your weekly and yearly programme (if you are a teacher); within your session (if you are a 'storyteller'); and in your family life for parents/carers.

If you find yourself always telling or reading the same type of story (e.g. always humorous, or always real, or always sad) then I suggest you try to stretch your tastes a little and look further for some new and different 'polarities', as your personality may be dominating your selection. With my love of Africa and African tales, I have to constantly remind myself to research and tell stories from other cultures!

Audience and venue

As a storyteller you will find yourself sifting through many stories until you find the ones that appeal – fortunately the story-well is bottomless! I strongly recommend that you love or at least like, or feel a connection to, the stories you choose to tell. However, it is equally important to take the audience into account when choosing a story or stories. Is the audience mono-cultural or multi-cultural, all boys or all girls, or mixed? Have the audience been involved already in hours of concentrated activity, or have they just arrived at school? Has your audience previously experienced 'told' stories (rather than read)?

If you are telling a story at a fair or festival, how much background noise and action may distract your listeners? For a noisy venue, you would be wise to plan stories with audience participation and lots of change and activity, rather than long and serious stories that require a high degree of concentration.

The age of the children, as discussed in a previous section, is also a significant factor, and your decisions here can be guided by common sense. I once read about an eminent actor sharing passages of 'Hamlet' with infant children and being surprised that the class quickly grew bored. Perhaps if he wanted to share Shakespeare, some light passages from Puck in 'A Midsummer Night's Dream' might have been a better choice for young ones, and even then it would be difficult to hold their concentration for long. Equally inappropriate would be telling 'The Gingerbread Man' to eleven-year-olds, unless you were preparing them to script a pantomime for little children.

Mixed-age audience

Sometimes a storyteller who is not connected as a teacher to a particular class is expected to tell stories to a mixed group, aged say between 4 and 9, at the library, or in a small school where the entire infants' department gathers to listen.

The best way to prepare for this is to choose some universal stories that are suited to a range of ages – a really good story, more often than not, is a good story for everyone. Such stories would need a 'happy ending' to ensure that the young ones' needs are considered, but could also be longer or more complex, or with humour, to appeal to the older ones. I have found that younger children seem to be able to concentrate for longer if the older children around them are absorbed in the story. The younger ones seem to imitate the 'concentration' level.

A tip for the times when you may have only a few older ones and mostly young ones is to tell stories for the younger audience but say to the older children before you begin: 'Here is a chance for you to learn a story to use when you are next babysitting younger children.' This will relieve the tension of older children feeling like 'babies'. If possible involve the older ones as helpers – holding the felt-board or playing the drum, etc.

Impromptu storytelling

Storytelling is not always such a planned experience. You will find that the more you enjoy sharing stories, the more occasions seem to pop up for you to do this, from babysitting a friend's child to being at a local restaurant with a group of friends.

As a teacher you may need to fill in ten minutes on an excursion while your class waits in a bus shelter for the bus; or you may have been asked to take a younger class while their teacher makes a phone call – the only way to be prepared for such impromptu events is to have a varied range of stories to draw on.

As a parent, there are unlimited possibilities for impromptu storytelling. In the car, at bedtime, on long walks, at the table while drawing a picture or doodling, in the kitchen while rolling the pastry or kneading dough (perhaps the Gingerbread Man can be replaced by a pastry or dough-ball man?). There are also rich possibilities in shared story banter, incorporating ideas from the children as you go along. In so many ways, families have the most fertile ground for planting and nurturing storytelling seeds.

In the professional environment, with a therapist or counsellor, opportunities for impromptu stories will arise with every new child. Stories or story ideas can be semi-prepared based on items in a story bag or box (with props and puppets inside), or items in a sand tray with animals and figurines. However, you may find it necessary to tell stories that take the needs of the individual child into account. Improvisation will be called for here.

30

Props and Presentation Ideas

Why use props?

Especially for young children, storytelling sessions can be enriched and extended by the use of props or presentation aids. The possibilities are endless, but it can help to keep your planning simple, for two main reasons:

1. The simpler the props the more the children's imaginations are left free to do the 'work'
2. The simpler the props the less preparation for the teller (an important consideration for a busy teacher, therapist or parent)

Children's imaginations can easily accept an open seedpod as a boat in the 'Magic Fish'; three gum-nuts or acorns as the three pigs and a pine cone as the wolf or hyena in the 'Three Little Pigs'; a large smooth stone for the hippo in the story of 'Hot Hippo'; or some knotted handkerchief dolls for a prince and princess.

I encourage you to experiment with simple ideas – you will be surprised how easy and effective they can be. Investigating story-telling in other cultures will provide inspiration here, for example:

- the use of 'picture cloths' in India
- the use of 'picture scrolls' in parts of Europe
- using storyboards in Papua New Guinea
- using folded paper figures in Japan
- working with string figures in parts of Asia, Africa and the Pacific
- sand drawings used in storytelling by indigenous Australian peoples
- working with song, dance and instruments (many cultures)

Many years ago at the local playgroup, when I first 'put down the book' and attempted to tell 'Goldilocks and the Three Bears', I was a nervous wreck of a human being! Having props was essential for me to get through the ordeal. I had arranged on the floor a little table with 3 bowls, 3 chairs (made from toy blocks), and 3 beds (made from little boxes). In my hand I clutched, at different times during the story, one doll and 3 different-sized bears, all found in the playgroup toy box. The props were set out in front of me so that by the time I had worked my way across the scenes, I would get through the story and the sequence would be correct. Eventually I reached the end. The children in front of me, oblivious to my nervous state, were sitting wide-eyed and asking for another story!

Many years later, I no longer need presentation aids to boost my confidence, but I still choose to use them sometimes (on a rare occasion even when telling stories to teenagers or adults) for the following reasons. Props can help …

- arouse curiosity
- the children to listen and concentrate
- the teller to remember the sequence of the story
- develop the confidence of a new storyteller
- add an artistic dimension to the story
- provide a variety of story presentations

To 'prop' or not to 'prop'?

Some stories lend themselves to the use of props – especially many of the short sequential and repetitive stories for young children, e.g. 'The Enormous Turnip and The Magic Fish'. Other stories are made more wondrous and magical with just one simple prop, e.g. cutting an apple across the middle to reveal the star inside adds a vital dimension to 'The Star Apple' story (see page 104). Playing a small drum throughout 'The Invisible Hunter' (see page 181), an American Indian fairytale, helps give strength to the repetitive song. Also, because it is quite a long story, the 'prop' of the song combined with the drumming can help keep audience concentration.

Even though props are more suited for use with storytelling for the younger age groups, don't discount their value for any age audience. I recently used a broom from the corner of the stage as a prop at an adult storytelling evening – it helped inject some necessary humour into the occasion!

Workability of props

Stories that are longer, with a more involved plot, are usually too complicated for props. A major production would be required, and this crosses into the realms of puppetry or theatre. It is usually simpler to let these stories unfold in the listener's imagination. Props could spoil this, and interrupt the concentration that develops during the storytelling process.

You also need to weigh up how much time you are prepared to spend on this. Whatever props you choose to make or use, they must be 'workable', i.e. not fall over, or not so many that you can't move them with two hands. You also need to practise with them several times before the 'performance'. A certain amount of 'choreography' and 'stage-sense' is needed here – e.g. not having the puppet or doll with its back to the audience, how to move it out of its house and across the scene, how (if the figure represents a person) to walk it like a human being and not 'hop it' like a kangaroo (and vice versa).

Over time you will develop a sense, through trial and error, of when a story needs props and when it works fine, or is stronger, without any help. Also you will know when you need props as a teller, and when you can do without.

My suggestion, especially if you are lacking confidence, is to start with props.

Different ways to 'prop' the same story

Some stories are not only well suited to the use of presentation aids, but can be 'propped' in many different ways (not all at once of course). In presenting the Norwegian tale of 'The Three Billy Goats', I have sat in a chair with a log on my lap (for the bridge) and a blue cloth flowing down to the floor (for the water). For the goats I have used stuffed knitted animals, or more simply, some teased white fleece or folded leaves. The troll can be represented by a knotted mess of dark-brown fleece, or a pinecone.

Alternatively, a puppet show can be set up on a table or in a sand tray, with some natural materials to create the scene, and some small knitted or clay animals for the characters. The story can also be told using a felt board, with felt pieces as props, or with finger puppets on one hand, and the other hand used as the bridge.

I have sometimes dressed children as the characters, using headbands with different-sized feathers for the billy-goat horns, and a large hooded cloak for the troll (who usually sits inside a basket next to me, and pops out at the right moments in the story). The 'goats' cross a bridge made from a long bench or a large log.

Another approach has been to 'prop' the story with musical instruments. For this I give all the children in the audience a range of different instruments for the characters – e.g. triangles or bells for the little goat; tambourines for the middle goat; drums for the large goat. Of course they have to learn to follow the storyteller / conductor, watching for when my hands lift up (to play) and go down (to stop).

All the above suggestions, and more (the possibilities are endless), can be experimented with and applied to many stories. Using props can be creative, enjoyable and fun for both the storyteller and the children!

Guidelines for Assessment of a Storytelling Session

Elements of Competence	Performance Criteria	Comments
1. Prepare storytelling situation	• Organise listeners to be in close sight and hearing of the teller • Prepare 'telling' space/chair • Prepare and set out any presentation aids (not essential) and have them within easy reach of storyteller	
2. Commence story	• Use technique(s) to gain the listeners' attention (e.g. sing a song, play music) • Create a mood of interest at the start	
3. Tell story	• Use suitable body language and gestures • Speak clearly • Speak in a 'flowing' way • Use a style of telling to suit the story and the age group of children (not too strong for the little ones) • Use pacing and spacing (i.e. not too fast or slow) • If using different voices for characters (not essential), ensure these voices are appropriate and don't get them confused	

		• Careful not to (over-)exaggerate characters, especially with very young children • Careful not to overload with descriptive language	
4. Conclude story		• Use technique(s) to end the storytelling session (e.g. sing, play music or a game)	
5. Holistic approach		• Be adequately prepared • Feel 'at home' with the story • Aim for a feeling of satisfaction in the story as a unit i.e. right length – not too long; not leaving the listeners wanting more detail. • 'Hold' the audience – i.e. weave that storytelling spell !	

Assessment: Competent .... Not yet competent ....

Comments:

31

Guidelines for Assessing Storytelling

The chart overleaf (see pages 270–271) has been used in formal storytelling courses to assess the skills of the teller. You may find it useful to print out and use as a way to evaluate yourself or others. Please don't be overwhelmed by this. Storytelling is personal and individual. Many natural storytellers have never submitted themselves to such an exercise.

The chart is included to help identify and clarify various 'elements of competence' in storytelling. It is probably more useful for teachers than parents.

However, a caution to all storytellers: when telling stories to young children, be careful not to exaggerate characters or use an over-dramatic telling style, especially for folk- or fairytales. This is a common mistake. Our aim should not be to scare or over-excite our young listeners but to nourish and strengthen them through the story's content. Trust in the power of the images to convey the story. Our main role as tellers to young children is simply to pass the story on to them. Their vivid imaginations will do the work all the better if our own personality does not overwhelm them.

32

Conclusion: A Story a Day

A story a day keeps the doctor away

If this book has achieved its aim then you will already be experiencing the medicinal qualities of 'a story a day'. After three decades of story experiences, I am still regularly surprised by their healing powers. Old stories continually come alive in different ways, while new stories bring fresh light into my life and work.

I was recently on a car journey with my eldest son and his little boy. The child was extremely upset as his mother had gone to work and he wanted to go with her. He was crying and squirming in his car seat, seemingly inconsolable. My son was upset because his child was upset, and I was sitting in the front seat wondering what I could say or do that could help. Then we turned a corner in the road, and Kieren's pile of surfboards in the back of the car slid across each other and made several loud squeaky noises. It reminded me of the 'squeaky bed' story, so I decided to tell it. My decision was a gamble, as little Tosh was quite young (he had only turned three that week) and he was making so much noise that at first my words could hardly be heard. Then suddenly, and magically, there was complete silence. Five minutes later I finished the story and a little voice said, 'Can we have 'nother one?' By the time we reached our destination, the three of us were singing songs and laughing and the mood had completely changed.

A difficult situation had, in the most simple and unplanned way, been healed by the power of 'story'.

*

A new story that has recently touched my life was from a Canadian colleague, Sandra, now living and working in Australia. A few weeks after attending one of my workshops, she contacted me to discuss her sudden and humbling task of helping plan a ceremony for a young child, a girl from her kindergarten who – a few months before her fourth birthday – had died from a snake-bite while camping in the rainforest with her family (see story on page 240).

Taking ideas from the parents, images from the rainforest and the child's other favourite things, and images from current natural phenomena (a comet passed overhead the day the child died), Sandra combined these with her own personal knowledge of the little girl, Shalem, and created a very moving ritual and story to share at the ceremony.

Shalem was described by many who knew her as 'a most ethereal little girl – a butterfly who fluttered here and there, a child with a lively imagination and an exuberant nature'. Shalem was close to her grandfather whom she thought was like a big Koala Bear. Some of Shalem's favourite things were playing 'peek-a-boo', being in nature, the colour blue, butterflies, insects, and bowerbirds (Australian birds that build bowers in the forest and love to decorate them with all things 'blue'). The morning after Shalem's death a bowerbird dropped a pair of blue plastic angel wings outside Shalem's family tent.

Sandra, on suggestion from the mother, chose the blue *Ulysses* butterfly as the metaphor in her story to represent the child and her journey. Called 'Shimmer Wing', it is about nature and life cycles, and builds a connection from the earth to the heavens. At the ceremony, Sandra invited all the children and adults gathered in front of her to help make the sounds of the rainforest at special times through the story, giving the story ritual a lighter quality. At the end, families were given a birdwing vine to take home and plant in their own gardens – in the story the yellow-bell flower from the 'birdwing' vine is Shimmer Wing's best friend.

Sandra's story is a beautiful example of how story making and storytelling worked together to help commemorate the tragic end of a young child's life. After Shalem's death her parents reported that her big brother seemed to be filled with a strength of character, a bravery that he had not had previously, as though his sister's courageous spirit had entered him. Shalem's best friend, Bethanni, was particularly attached to a toy unicorn after her death. Bethanni's mother commented how intently her daughter listened to the story at the ceremony.

There were other stories of individual growth following Shalem's death and the ceremony. Shalem's parents were very grateful for Sandra's contribution and commented that 'no wonder Shalem thought of Sandra as her 'fairy godmother' and loved coming to her kindergarten'. Apparently Shalem would not settle at any other daycare centre, and her mother had to keep searching until Shalem and Sandra found each other.

*

One of the most satisfying outcomes of my work with healing stories has been the growing network of workshop participants who send their thoughts, questions and story ideas to me. Most of these come via email, but some, particularly from many African colleagues, come across the ocean in text messages from their mobile phones.

Susan, need help with story for boy – 6 years – always pushing – too rough for others in group – any ideas?

Text messages pose an interesting problem for me if I want to write several 'paragraphs' in reply:

How about a story with a warthog that has to learn to use his tusks to do constructive things – like dig for food, dig holes to live in – perhaps start with warthog losing friends because of hurting them all the time with his strong tusks – then warthog comes across someone/something in need – perhaps stuck in mud – warthog helps him out and gains a friend – what do you think?

Fortunately I have recently mastered the art of using 'predictive text'. Even better news is that some of my African colleagues now have computers and we can send long emails back and forth. Occasionally I call and attempt to chat over a crackling line.

The other night I opened my 'inbox' and found the following email from an Australian childcare worker.

I have attended a few of your workshops, the most recent in April this year. You mentioned it would be OK to write to you. I run a Steiner-influenced family daycare service and look after 3- to 5-year-olds.

Attached is a story – 'The Monkey Tree'. I wrote it for a four-year-old child in my care whose parents separated last year. The child was finding it difficult adapting to new, shared custody arrangements. She has 3 teenage siblings and her home life is often noisy and a little 'chaotic', which is why I chose the monkey theme.

I would very much welcome your comments and feedback. Hoping I am on the right track. I have gained such a lot from your workshops and even write healing stories for myself!

I then opened the attachment and had the privilege of reading a beautifully written story – simple, with great repetition and rhyme suitable for a four-year-old, and excellent use of the framework of 'metaphor, journey and resolution' to meet the challenging situation.

In my reply I gushed positive feedback, then asked the following questions, which are vital for evaluating any therapeutic story:

Since telling the story have you observed any change in the behaviour of the child and family?

How many times have you told it at your daycare centre?

Have you given the story to the parents/grandparents/other carers to share with the child? If so, do you have any feedback from this?

A day later, her reply comprehensively answered the above questions:

'Z' has been in my care since February 2006. 'Z' was clearly quite upset and lacking confidence during the initial separation of her parents last year, but she eventually settled, although I could see her confidence was still low with the other children. When the new custody arrangements were made this year, she started to regress and become anxious and would cry and get upset when her parents left, and on occasion became very distressed.

That was when I decided to write the story. I gave the story to her mother to read at home and noticed an improvement at daycare almost immediately. I understand she often goes home to mum during her time with dad, but she has settled completely again with us here in daycare and is more confident and happier than at any time over the past year-and-a-half. I have spoken to her mum who says she read the story a few times and that 'Z' occasionally mentions the 'Monkey Tree', so seems to remember it. Mum also notes that she has become far less clingy and demanding and in fact is now the least emotionally demanding of the four children. I recently sent mum a photo, as her smile was more natural and real than I have seen for a long time.

With Jilly's permission, I felt honoured to include 'The Monkey Tree' in this book (see page 246).

More recently, my email network seems to be magically growing to include people I have never met, from lands I have not yet visited. This morning, I opened a 'gem' from Whitehorse near the Alaskan border.

I have purchased some of your healing story collections presented to me by a kindergarten teacher from New Zealand. I now tell some of your stories regularly in my early childhood programs here in the Yukon in Canada, close to Alaska. For me they are my most valuable stories and the children are always touched by them in a special way.

I would love to attend one of your workshops and would like to know when and where you will have workshops in North America.

From this, plans are developing to visit the Yukon next year, with an open invitation for my husband and me to stay with this new 'online' friend. The arrangement is to exchange stories and story workshops for accommodation and meals. I have since been informed that her husband's business is an organic bakery. 'A story a day' could mean that we will probably eat too much and need 'a long walk a day'!

And a long walk a day may help bring new ideas for stories. While walking through the valleys and listening to the winds blow across the Yukon mountains, who knows what stories I may hear.

*

As this book comes full circle, I want to end it with a story.

Entitled 'Lindelwe's Song', it is one I wrote many years ago about a 'magic pumpkin'. I presented it as a gift to the women who were attending my training courses in South Africa in 1997. Its metaphors, journey and resolution were inspired by the following comment once made to me by an African friend, Nomangesi Mzamo.

Without our singing we would never have found our way through the thorns of apartheid.

It has since found its way into many Educare Centres and schools in the Cape Town townships. A friend, Nombulelo Majesi, once described it as a healing story for the new South Africa.

I always thought that this story had its main place and purpose in Africa. When I visit both Cape Town and Kenya, children and adults whom I meet and work with ask for it again and again – some of the children have given me the nickname 'The pumpkin lady'.

However, I should have known better than to think that a story could be restricted to one 'place' and 'purpose'. This year, to my surprise, it was presented as a puppet show at the recent 'Vital Years', an Australian biennial national early childhood conference. A friend called me about it, and then told me she was planning to return home (to the sub-tropical coast of north-eastern Australia) and present a similar puppet show for her school's open day. These were her comments emailed to me after the event:

Hi Susan,
Just to let you know 'Lindelwe' was appreciated on many levels, from grandparents to toddlers. The atmosphere was spell-binding and magical. The metaphors you used are relevant to everyone, regardless of which country we live in. We will do a repeat performance this Thursday for the year 12 students followed by one for the teachers.. Thanks again.
Regards,
Carol G – 4.8.07

Lindelwe's Song

Once upon a time, in the middle of a field next to a village, a tiny pumpkin seed started to grow. It grew and it grew and it grew – until its green vines covered the ground, and in the middle of the pumpkin patch was the biggest and most beautiful golden pumpkin that the villagers had ever seen.

But this was no ordinary pumpkin, and this was no ordinary field. As the pumpkin was growing, a circle hedge of thorn bushes grew up around the pumpkin patch. These bushes were so close and thick with thorns that by the time the pumpkin was ripe and ready to be picked, no one could get through the hedge to get to it.

The villagers had a meeting to decide what could be done. At the meeting an old grandfather said: 'I have a sharp axe – I will try to chop down the hedge of thorns.' So he took his sharp axe and started to chop through the hedge, but every time he chopped through a branch, another grew quickly in its place, and by the end of the day he had given up.

Then one of the mothers of the village said: 'I have a strong spade – I will try to dig under the hedge of thorns.' So she took her spade and started to dig down, but the roots of the thorn bushes were so strong and close together that by the end of the day she too had given up.

Then one of the young boys of the village said: 'I am such a good tree climber – I will try to climb over the hedge of thorns.' So he started to climb up the branches, but the thorns were as long and sharp as needles and they tore his clothes and pricked his skin, and by the end of the day he too had given up.

The next day Lindelwe, a young girl known to have the most beautiful voice in all the land, walked through the village. When she heard the problem she walked past the villagers, sat down on a rock next to the hedge of thorns, and started to sing:

Ithanga elikulu, Ithanga elikulu; lishleli ebobeni, lishleli ebobeni

Lindelwe's singing was so beautiful that all the animals in the surrounding fields came closer to listen. [Repeat song]

Lindelwe's singing was so beautiful that the birds in the sky flew down to sit in the trees to listen. [Repeat song]

Lindelwe's singing was so beautiful that the worms and caterpillars crawled out of the ground to sit at her feet to listen. [Repeat song]

Lindelwe's singing was so beautiful that even the clouds in the sky came down low to listen. [Repeat song]

One little cloud came so low that it landed right in front of her. Lindelwe stopped singing and smiled at the watching villagers as she stepped onto the middle of the little cloud. And the cloud lifted her up and over the hedge of thorns and right into the middle of the pumpkin patch.

And there, Lindelwe was able to pick the beautiful pumpkin and carry it back onto the little cloud. And the little cloud then lifted her up and over the hedge of thorns and all the way back to the centre of the village.

The villagers cooked the pumpkin for an enormous feast that evening. At the feast they celebrated the day that Lindelwe, with her beautiful singing, was able to find a way over the magic hedge of thorns to pick the most wonderful, most golden pumpkin in the land.

Appendix 1

Recommended books and websites

BOOKS

Barfield, O. (1977), *Matter, Imagination and Spirit – The Rediscovery of Meaning and Other Essays,* Wesleyan University Press: Middletown, CT

Baldwin Dancy, Rahima (2006), *You Are Your Child's First Teacher,* Hawthorn Press, Stroud

Barton, B. (1991), *Tell Me Another,* Rigby Heinemann, Victoria.

Bettelheim, B. (1976), *The Uses of Enchantment,* Penguin Books, Middlesex, England.

Blaxland-de Lange, S. (2006), *Owen Barfield: A Biography,* Temple Lodge: U.K.

Cassady, M. (1990) *Storytelling Step By Step,* Resource Publ., California

Dodd, S. (1994), *Managing Problem Behaviours,* MacLennan & Petty Pty Ltd, NSW

Edmunds, L. Francis (2004), *Introduction to Steiner Education: The Waldorf School,* Rudolf Steiner Press, Sussex

Egan, K. (1988). *Teaching as Storytelling,* Routledge, London

Estes, C.P. (1992), *Women who run with the Wolves,* Rider, London

Gersie, A. (1991). *Storymaking in Bereavement,* Jessica Kingsley Publishers, London.

Greer, C. & Kohl, H. (1995) *A Call to Character: A Family Treasury of Stories, Poems, Plays, Proverbs and Fables,* Harper Collins, N.Y.

Groome, H. (1994), *Teaching Aboriginal Studies Effectively,* Social Science Press, Sydney.

Johnston, A. (1996), *Eating in the Light of the Moon,* Birch Lane Press, N.J.

Kilpatrick,W. & Wolfe,G.(1994), *Books That Build Character – A Guide to Teaching your Child Moral Values through Storytelling,* Touchstone, N.Y.

Mani, G. (1996) *Storyteller, Storyteacher: Discovering the Power of Story Telling for Teaching and Living,* Stenhouse, York.

McDonald, M. R. (1993) *The Storytellers' Start-up Book,* August House, Little Rock, Arkansas.

McKay, H. & Dudley, B. (1996) *About Storytelling: A Practical Guide,* Hale & Iremonger, Sydney

Mellon, N. (1992). *Storytelling and the Art of Imagination,* Element, Dorset

Mellon, N. (2000). *Storytelling with Children,* Hawthorn Press, Stroud

Meyer, R. (1981), *The Wisdom of Fairy Tales*, Floris Books, Edinburgh

Milne, A.A. (1973), *When We Were Very Young* and *Now We Are Six,* Methuen: London

Okri, B. (1996), *Birds of Heaven,* Phoenix, London

Pearmain, E.D. (2006), *Once Upon a Time: Storytelling to Teach Character and Prevent Bullying,* Marco Products, PA.

Pellowski, A.(1990), *The World of Storytelling,* H.W. Wilson Company, N.Y.

Porter, L. (1999), *Young Children's Behaviour: Practical Approaches for Caregivers and Teachers,* MacLennan & Petty Pty Ltd, NSW

Steiner, R. (2001), *Nature Spirits – Selected Lectures,* Translated by M. Barton, Rudolf Steiner Press, London

Steiner, R. (1989) *The Poetry and Meaning of Fairy Tales,* Mercury Press, N.Y.

Van der Post, L. (1972), *'A Story Like The Wind',* Penguin Books, London.

Watson, M. 1986, *'To Spear a Hotdog – Storytelling for Today's Children',* in *Coming Out!* Nelson, Vic.

Wyatt, I. (1975), *The Seven-Year-Old Wonder Book,* Dawn-Leigh Publications, CA.

WEBSITES

Healing Story Alliance
http://www.healingstory.org/
The purpose of this alliance is to explore and promote storytelling for healing by sharing story experiences and skills.

World-Wide Storytelling Studies
http://courses.unt.edu/efiga/STORYTELLING/WorldWideList. htm

Information on storytelling training around the world

Susan Perrow
http://healingthroughstories.com/
A website to encourage dialogue on writing therapeutic stories and to promote Susan Perrow's storybooks.

Storytelling Unit – Southern Cross University
http://www.scu.edu.au/schools/edu/
Unit Code: ENG00355

Nancy Mellon's Website
http://www.healingstory.com/
Information on international storytelling events and Nancy's School of Therapeutic Storytelling

Elisa Pearmain
http://wisdomtales.com/character/
Once Upon a Caring Classroom: storytelling for character education and bullying prevention in the K-8 classroom.

Indigenous Peoples Literature
http://www.indigenouspeople.net/
Central site for indigenous literature (worldwide) – many links available from this – a wealth of stories and cultural collections

Storyarts
http://www.storyarts.org
Includes ideas for storytelling in the classroom, lesson plans and activities for storytelling across the curriculum, and audio samples of Heather Forest's musical stories.

Stories for the Seasons
http://www.h-net.org/~nilas/seasons/
Offers seasonal and nature stories (for ages 5-12) together with an extensive bibliography on stories of animals and plants.

Storytelling and Arts Empowerment

http://www.artslynx.org/heal/stories.htm
The resources on this website allow you to explore how the story-telling arts are used to build strong individuals and communities

Karen Chase
http://www.storybug.net/links.htm
http://www.storybug.net/pdf/stories_a_to_z.pdf
There are unlimited resources on these sites – full text of folktales from all over the world, full set of Rudyard Kipling's stories, puppetry sites through to interactive story resources – a year's worth of reading!

Tales of Wonder
http://www.darsie.net/talesofwonder/
An archive of folk- and fairytales. The stories in this collection represent a small sample of the rich storytelling heritage. Stories from many parts of the world are included here.

Story Lovers Website
http://www.story-lovers.com/index.html
A celebration of the world's best loved stories and rhymes PLUS a comprehensive archival library for finding stories, sources and advice from professional storytellers

Collection of Grimms Tales
http://www.cs.cmu.edu/~spok/grimmtmp/
Complete text of 209 tales based on the translation by Margaret Hunt, called Grimm's Household Tales

Wonder Homeschool
http://www.wonderhs.com/
Stories and other resources for parents who are home schooling – great ideas for teachers too!

Imaginative Education Research Group
http://www.ierg.net/
This site belongs to a group of researchers, teachers, graduate students, parents, and others who would like to make education more

effective. They call their new approach 'Imaginative Education' (IE) because engaging students' imaginations in learning, and teachers' imaginations in teaching, seems crucial to making knowledge in the curriculum vivid and meaningful to students. The IERG was founded in 2001 at the Faculty of Education at Simon Fraser University, British Columbia, Canada.

Spirit of Trees Website
http://www.spiritoftrees.org/
A resource for therapists, educators, environmentalists, storytellers and tree lovers. Here you will find a varied collection of multicultural folktales and myths that relate to trees.

Australian Dreamtime Stories
http://www.dreamtime.net.au/
A wonderful resource for storytellers and teachers. The site explores indigenous Australia through storytelling, cultures and histories. It includes Stories of the Dreaming, teachers' resources and content for students.

The Flowering Tree and other Indian Tales
http://ark.cdlib.org/ark:/13030/ft067n99wt/
A collection of oral tales by A.K. Ramanujan

The Story Vine
http://www.drawandtell.com/hastoryvine.html
An online collection of draw-and-tell sand stories, plus stories for storytelling, writing ideas and language activities.

Anansi Stories
http://www.robinsononeil.com/anansi_folk_tales.htm
An online collection of both the Caribbean and African Anansi stories

Kid's Storytelling Club
http://www.storycraft.com
Resources for helping children become storytellers, ideas for storytelling aids, presentation skills, etc.

Oral Tradition Journal
http://journal.oraltradition.org/
Oral Tradition is an international and interdisciplinary forum for the discussion of worldwide oral traditions and related forms.
The journal is now available electronically at:
http://journal.oraltradition.org and free of charge to all readers

Kim-John Payne, M.Ed
http://www.thechildtoday.com/
Kim Payne is a counsellor, researcher and educator, who works on issues of social difficulties amongst siblings and classmates, attention and behavioural challenges at home and school, and emotional problems such as defiance, aggression, addiction and self-esteem.

Alliance for Childhood
http://www.allianceforchildhood.org/
A worldwide organisation that promotes policies and practices that support children's healthy development, love of learning, and joy in living. Their public education campaigns in many countries bring to light both the promise and the vulnerability of childhood. They act for the sake of the children themselves and for a more just, democratic, and ecologically responsible future. Lists many links, resources and current publications.

Resource Unit for Children with Special Needs, Inc:
http://www.rucsn.org.au/
Established in 1987, its primary role is to enable children with special needs to be included in childcare facilities in Western Australia. Its website offers excellent resources, fact sheets etc. on a wide range of behaviour disorders and challenging behaviours.

Early Childhood Australia
http://www.earlychildhoodaustralia.org.au/
Offers resources, newsletters, fact sheets etc. on child development and most early childhood topics

NSW Government

– Dept of Community Services Parenting Site
http://www.community.nsw.gov.au/html/parenting/parenting.htm
Offers resources, newsletters, fact sheets etc. on parenting issues and topics.

Parent Shop Resources
http://www.parentshop.com.au/
Helping parents increase their competency with easy-to-use and effective parenting (& teaching) resources.

Jenni Cargill – Australian Storyteller
& Director of The Storytree Company
http://www.thestorytreecompany.com.au
Offers a wealth of storytelling training, performances and resources – based at Byron Bay, NSW.

My Magical Story Journal
http://www.storyspeaks.com.au/
This Australian website and related book is a tool to help create therapeutic stories for children and to enrich the imaginative powers of adults – a treasure chest for teachers, parents, relatives, friends and carers.

Appendix 2

Completed story charts

See pages 290-6 for a suggested completion of Tables One and Two from Chapter Five (pages 68-71).

Table One: ANALYSING THERAPEUTIC STORIES – General types of behaviour

STORY	METAPHOR(S)	JOURNEY	RESOLUTION
Tembe's Boots (page 118)	• Little red boots • 'Friends together'	• A description (with much repetition) of the daily adventures of a pair of boots	• Boots taken off feet and put carefully together at rest-time, not thrown in a messy pile
The Grandmother and the Donkey (page 123)	• Nature's child • Grandmother • Donkey • Seeds / flowers • Litter in streets • Loss of connection to nature	• Moving from the country to the town • Moving from beauty to ugliness and back to beauty	• Children helping to clean up the litter and plant gardens
Little Straw Broom (page 220)	• Little people (used as puppets) • Coloured hats • Repetition and rhyme	• Three little men take turns using the broom • One couldn't be bothered, one is too fast and wild, one is careful and committed to the task	• Gold hat shows how to sweep crumbs into a pile • Broom satisfied it has done a good job

Restless Red Pony (page 199)	• Wild pony • Farmer • Grooming brush • Song	• Pony slowly learns to stop kicking wildly all the time and enjoys keeping still to be touched and groomed	• Friends sharing together • A positive experience of being still and being cared for • Careful touching as opposed to hitting and kicking
Whingeing (Whining) Whale (page 100)	• Whale pod • Whinge song • Whale song • Reef • Shallow water	• Young whale so busy whingeing loses his way and gets caught in shallow lagoon; he is rescued by his use of whale song	• Whingeing replaced by more constructive uses of voice • Feeling of belonging • Joy of singing
Impatient Zebra (page 146)	• Brown stripes • vBlack stripes • Shade / sun • Reflection	• Young zebra moping around – wants to have black stripes like the older zebras – tries different ways to turn his brown stripes into black ones	• It takes time to grow • Sometimes waiting is important • You can't hurry development • Eating and playing help growth

Table Two: ANALYSING THERAPEUTIC STORIES – Specific Situations

STORY	METAPHOR(S)	JOURNEY	RESOLUTION
Baby Bear Koala (page 249)	• Tree (world) • Hungry growing baby • Tired mother • Juicy leaves • Higher branches	• Mother and baby in tree, mother falls asleep, hungry baby climbs by himself to reach juicy leaves	• Young koala becomes strong enough and brave enough to leave mother and venture into the world by himself
Cranky Crab (page 159)	• Nippers • Unhappy beach friends • Wise tortoise • Knitted mittens	• Crab unpopular as he is always hurting others with his nippers – tortoise knits crab some mittens to keep his nippers warm and cosy and out of the way	• Learning to use nippers/hands in non-hurting ways • Inclusive solution for dealing with hurting behaviour
The Pocket Knife and the Castle (page 119)	• 'Singing' pocket knife • Castle • Dream • Silver moonlight	• Repetition of destructive 'cutting' and its consequences, followed by a dream and the carving of a wooden castle	• Boy experiences the joy of creating something beautiful • Motivation to use hands and tools to construct rather than destroy or damage

Born to be King (page 230)	• Prince • Broken bones • Castle walls • Wise woman • Grandma's mirror • Sunlight • Dark room • Crown as prop	• Accident and slow healing process • Light to dark to light • Outside to inside to outside	• Prince needs to walk out into the sunlight by himself • Building of self-confidence and inner strength
Cloud Boy Story (page 22)	• Boy who lived in the clouds • Doll as a prop	• 'Cloud Boy' makes his way down to live in the world	• Child bonds with and cares for new doll • Influence of peer group and commercial doll transformed
The Towel Story (page 192)	• Grandfather towel • New little towel • Song	• Learning how to be a towel and learning the towel song	• New towel is happy because it has had a chance to be a 'towel' • Child has positive experience of standing still and being dried

Other Books from Hawthorn Press

Therapeutic Storytelling

Susan Perrow

Susan Perrow uses imaginative journeys and the magic of metaphor in her therapeutic storytelling to resolve children's challenging behaviour. This treasury of 101 new healing stories addresses a range of issues – from bullying, grieving, anxiety, nightmares, intolerance, bedwetting and much more. She offers a tried and tested method for creating a unique story for a child to help them build emotional resilience and character.

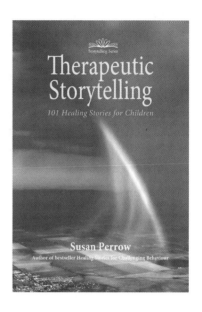

256pp;234 x 156mm; pb; 978-1-907359-15-6

An A-Z Collection of Behaviour Tales
From Angry Ant to Zestless Zebra

Susan Perrow

Susan offers story medicine as a creative strategy to help children age 3–9 years face challenges and change behaviour. Following the alphabet, each undesirable behaviour is identified in the story title: anxious, bullying, demanding, fussy, jealous, loud, obnoxious, uncooperative, and more. The stories, some humorous and some serious, are ideal for parenting, teaching and counselling.

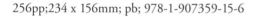

144pp; 234 x 156mm; pb; 978-1-907359-86-6

Stories to Light the Night

Susan Perrow

A unique, comprehensive collection of 94 imaginatively crafted stories for sharing with children, families and communities at times of grieving, bereavement, separation or loss. The stories come from different contributors and from many different cultures and countries worldwide. There are also Patterns and Templates for activities provided for some of the stories.

192pp; 234 x 156mm; pb; 978-1-912480-27-2

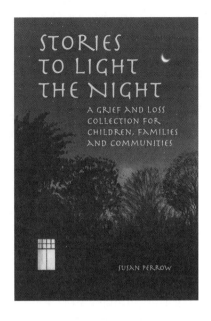

Storytelling with Children

Nancy Mellon

Telling stories is a peaceful, magical way of creating special occasions with children. Nancy believes every parent can, and should, become a confident, creative storyteller, and that stories told by a parent are a gift to your child, a wonderful act of sharing and communicating. Nancy's gentle, practical advice is illustrated with many beautiful, funny and wise stories created by families who have discovered how the power of story transforms lives and relationships.

192pp; 216 × 138mm; pb; 978-1-907359-26-2

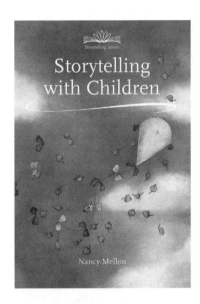

Raising Happy Healthy Children

Sally Goddard Blythe

This new title is a fully-updated second edition of Sally's previous book *What Children and Babies Really Need.* It presents convincing research to show how a baby's relationship with its mother has a lasting, deep impact. Recent social changes are interfering with key developmental milestones that are essential for wellbeing in later life. Sally Goddard Blythe says: 'We need a society that gives children their parents, and most of all values motherhood in the early years.'

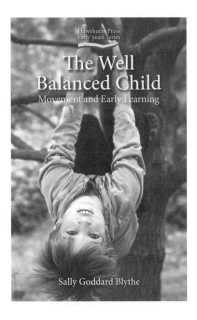

260pp; 234 x 156mm; pb; 978-1-907359-83-5

The Well Balanced Child

Sally Goddard Blythe

'Learning is not just about reading, writing and maths' says Sally. She believes a child's experience of movement plays a pivotal role in shaping their personality, feelings and achievements. This book makes the case for a 'whole body' approach to learning, which integrates the brain, senses, movement, music and play.

240pp; 216 x 138mm; pb; 978-1-903458-63-1

Free to Learn

Lynne Oldfield

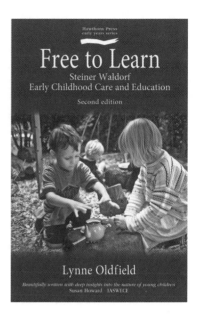

The belief of Steiner Waldorf kindergartens and childcare centres is that children's early learning is profound, that childhood matters, and that the early years should be enjoyed, not rushed through. Lynne draws on her extensive kindergarten experience from around the world, with stories, helpful insights, lively observations and vivid pictures.

240pp; 216 x 138mm; pb; 978-1-907359-13-2

Muddles, Puddles and Sunshine

Diana Crossley
Illustrated by
Kate Sheppard

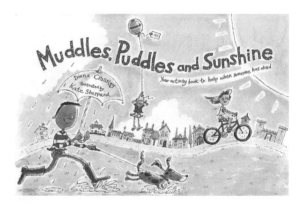

This book offers practical and sensitive support for bereaved children. Beautifully illustrated, it suggests a helpful series of activities and exercises, accompanied by the friendly characters of Bee and Bear. It gives a structure and an outlet for the many difficult feelings which inevitably follow when someone dies, and aims to help children make sense of their experience by reflecting on the different aspects of their grief, whilst finding a balance between remembering and having fun.

32pp; 297 × 210mm; pb; 978-1-869890-58-2

Jumping Mouse

Brian Patten
Illustrated by Mary Moore

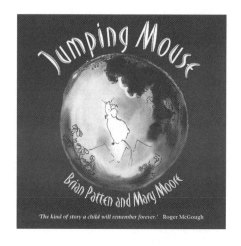

This Native American folk tale tells how a little mouse had the courage to leave his family's warm nest in the roots of a giant tree, and go in search of the Sacred Mountains. He has many adventures on the way and finds his true name of Jumping Mouse. This hero quest has enchanted generations of children since first publication in 1972. Brian Patten has updated his original version of the story for this second edition, which also reproduces the original illustrations by Mary Moore, the daughter of the sculptor Henry Moore.

48pp; 210 × 210mm; hb; 978-1-903458-99-0

Making the Children's Year
Seasonal Waldorf Crafts with Children

Marije Rowling

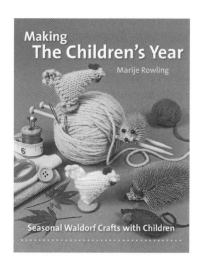

Bringing new inspiration and ideas to a modern readership, this book is packed with all kinds of crafts, from papercrafting to building dens. For beginners and experienced crafters, this book is a gift for parents and adults seeking to make toys that will inspire children and provide an alternative to our throwaway culture. Marije reminds us that making things by hand brings inner and outer rewards, and encourages joy in creating and in acknowledging the rhythms of the year.

240pp; 250 x 200mm; pb; 978-1-907359-69-9

Findus Plants Meatballs

Sven Nordqvist

Farmer Pettson begins to sow his vegetables and because Findus doesn't like vegetables he decides to plant one of his meatballs instead. However, keeping the vegetable garden safe from the farm animals proves a hard task for Findus and Pettson. Translated from Swedish, this is one of ten wonderful tales about an old man and his talking cat.

28pp; 297 × 210mm; hb; 978-1-907359-29-3

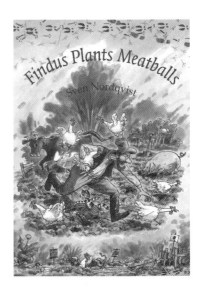

Findus, Food and Fun
Seasonal crafts and nature activities

Eva-Lena Larsson, Kennert Danielsson and Sven Nordqvist

Findus, Food and Fun is for mums, dads, grandparents, teachers, childminders, aunts, uncles and anyone who knows a young child who is curious about the world. Together with Findus, Pettson and the muckles, you can discover things to do for every season; pottering, collecting, fixing, crafting, building, exploring, baking. Sometimes outdoors, sometimes indoors, here is a whole year's worth of ideas.

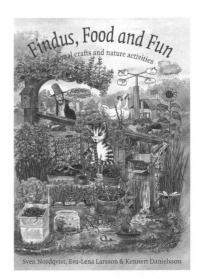

64pp; 297 x 210mm; hb; 978-1-907359-34-7

The Natural Storyteller

Georgiana Keable

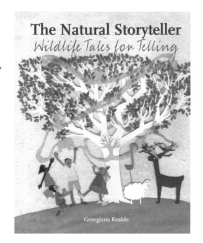

Here is a staggering wealth of both new and traditional stories all about nature and our role as humans in it. Culturally diverse and all told with great energy and panache, the stories will engage young readers and encourage them to become natural storytellers. The book includes storymaps and practical activities that can be undertaken individually or as a group.

272pp; 228 x 186mm; pb; 978-1-907359-80-4

The Case for Homeschooling

Seasonal crafts and nature activities

Anna Dusseau

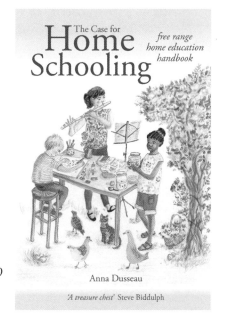

A must-read for families considering teaching their children at home. Alongside practical tips for getting started and answers to key questions, you will find a wealth of tried and tested activities. The informative, honest accounts of homeschooling show different approaches so as to help choices.

248pp; 234 × 156mm; pb; 978-1-912480-28-9

Ebook 978-1-912480-41-8

Ordering books

If you have difficulties ordering Hawthorn Press books from a bookshop,
you can order direct from our website:

www.hawthornpress.com

or from our UK distributor:

Booksource
50 Cambuslang Road, Glasgow, G32 8NB
Tel: (0845) 370 0063
E-mail: orders@booksource.net

Hawthorn Press

www.hawthornpress.com